Aids to Undergraduate Medicine

J. L. Burton

B.Sc., M.D., M.R.C.P.
Consultant Senior Lecturer in Dermatology
Bristol Royal Infirmary

Aids to Undergraduate Medicine

J. L. Burton

Second Edition

CHURCHILL LIVINGSTONE
EDINBURGH LONDON AND NEW YORK 1976

CHURCHILL LIVINGSTONE
Medical Division of Longman Group Limited

Distributed in the United States of America by Longman Inc., 19 West 44th Street, New York, N.Y. 10036, and by associated companies, branches and representatives throughout the world.

First Edition   1973
    Reprinted   1974
Second Edition   1976
    Reprinted   1977
    Reprinted   1979

ISBN 0 443 01502 3

Library of Congress Cataloging in Publication Data

Burton, John Lloyd.
    Aids to undergraduate medicine.

    Includes index.
    1. Medicine—Outlines, syllabi, etc.   I. Title.
[DNLM: 1. Medicine—Outlines.   W18 B974a]
RC58.B85   1976   616'.002'02   76-8509

Printed in Great Britain
by Bell and Bain Ltd., Glasgow

Preface to the Second Edition

In this edition many lists have been slightly modified to bring them up to date. The introductory section 'Hints on the Final M.B. Examination' has been expanded, and several new lists have been added in response to requests from students. These include sections on oral contraceptives, complications of myocardial infarction and the causes of coma, epilepsy, syncope, dysphagia, osteoporosis and osteomalacia.

1976   J. L. B.

Preface

This little book is primarily intended to provide a compact aid to revision for candidates taking the Final M.B. Medicine examination. My previous book, *Aids to Postgraduate Medicine*, which was intended for M.R.C.P. candidates, has apparently been used for revision by many undergraduate students and I hope this companion volume will prove more suited to their needs, though candidates for other medical examinations may also find it helpful.

Medical educators are unanimous in their condemnation of learning by rote. Nevertheless, candidates in medical examinations still find it necessary to retain a formidable number of facts and I believe that the use of 'skeleton' lists as an adjunct to comprehensive textbooks can encourage an orderly approach to the subject as well as provide a basis for expansion in answers to examination questions.

It is impossible to achieve comprehensive coverage in a book of this size, but I have tried to select information which is worth remembering for use either in the assessment of common clinical situations or in reply to some of the more commonly asked examination questions. Many of the lists I have included are not readily available in the usual undergraduate textbooks, and for some important examination topics I have provided lists which are more detailed than those given in most undergraduate textbooks. Doubtless some readers will be disappointed by the omission of a favourite list and, as a small measure of compensation, there are several blank pages to enable supplementary information to be added according to the personal preferences and needs of the individual.

Few of the lists in this book are original. Most have been derived from standard specialist texts or medical journals, and where modification has been necessary I accept responsibility for any errors which may have arisen. I should like to thank many of my friends and colleagues, too numerous to mention individually, who have given me much helpful advice and criticism.

1973   J. L. B.

Contents

Hints on the Final M.B.
Medicine Examination

> Examinations are formidable even to the best prepared,
> for the greatest fool may ask more than the wisest man
> can answer.
>
> Charles C. Colton (1820) *Lacon*, **I**, 322

The Final M.B. examination is intended to prevent the
qualification of incompetent doctors, and the examiners have
the duty of ensuring that every successful candidate is safe to be
'licensed to heal'. They require to know that:

(i) you have a sound knowledge of the basic principles of
     medicine and a common sense approach to the subject;
(ii) you've had practical experience on the wards and can
     detect and interpret physical signs;
(iii) you can prescribe safely, i.e. you know the mode of
      administration and approximate dosage of important
      drugs, and you know their main actions and serious
      side-effects;
(iv) you can recognize and treat medical emergencies
     competently.

Any candidate who satisfies the examiners on these points is
fairly certain to pass the examination, but bear in mind the
lugubrious corollary that if the examiners demonstrate a deficiency
in these abilities, failure may follow.

Revision
An important function of revision is to identify and eliminate
'blind spots'. Nobody can know everything, but you should aim
to be completely ignorant about nothing, and the commoner the
topic, the more you should know about it. A good way to cover
topics which are likely to occur in the examination is to see as
many cases on the wards as possible during your training and to
'read around' them. Most good physicians base their knowledge
on cases they have seen personally, and it's quite a good idea as
a student to keep a brief record of the patients you have seen as
an aid to later revision.

A sound knowledge of medicine is obviously essential, but
rapid recall of that knowledge in the exam is equally important.
Instead of reading part of the textbooks in detail just before
the exam, it's better to refresh your memory of the whole field,
even if only in a superficial way. This will be facilitated if your

1

lecture notes are all kept on loose-leaf paper of a standard size so that your knowledge from the various subspecialities can be integrated to avoid confusion and duplication of effort.

Essay questions

The purpose of an essay question is to discover whether you can assemble your knowledge of a subject, select appropriate facts and opinions, arrange them in an orderly manner and then express yourself with clarity and good style. You should ask yourself what the examiners are trying to test in a particular question. They often have a fairly rigid marking code, awarding marks for each of certain predetermined points that are made, and no extra marks are awarded for even the most fascinating digressions. Candidates rarely fail Final M.B. on the essay questions, but those who do are usually failed for not answering the questions that were asked.

Another cause for failure is misjudgement of the time allotted to each question. You should apply the 'Law of Diminishing Returns' as it applies to essay questions—the first 40 per cent for any question is easy, the next 30 per cent is much harder, the next 20 per cent is virtually impossible and the final 10 per cent *is* impossible. Consistency in every question should be your aim. You should not however waste too much time on a question which you cannot answer. A blank simply scores no marks but an effusion of rubbish will prejudice the examiner against you.

Where possible questions should be answered in terms of disturbance of physiology. This will demonstrate your knowledge of basic principles and also help you to arrange your answer in an orderly and rational manner.

Many candidates spend hours trying to predict questions by studying old papers. The syllabus is too big for this to be profitable in Final M.B., but it's worth checking the type of questions you'll be asked and spending time on any topics on which you are ignorant.

Multiple-choice questions

M.C.Q.s are here to stay and you should familiarize yourself with the type of question favoured by your own medical school, particularly since you may be faced with an instruction such as—

Each question below consists of an assertion (statement) and a reason. On the appropriate line of the answer sheet blacken the space under—

(a) if both assertion and reason are true and the reason is a correct explanation of the assertion,

(b) if both assertion and reason are true but the reason is not a correct explanation of the assertion,

(c) if the assertion is true but the reason is a false statement,

(d) if the assertion is false but the reason is a true statement,

(e) if both assertion and reason are false statements.

Many candidates worry about whether they will lose marks for guessing in M.C.Q. exams. It's true that the examiners can adjust scores for the effect of guessing, knowing the number of choices for each question and applying a corrective formula, but the usual correction deducts less than 1 mark for a wrong guess, so unless you are specifically instructed to the contrary it is worth attempting every question. In any case it is a rare question in which you cannot eliminate at least one 'false' answer and whenever you can you have a probability greater than chance of choosing the correct response. Remember too that the words 'always' and 'never' rarely apply to medicine and responses which contain them are unlikely to be true.

Another problem arises when a student has personally seen an unusual case which is the 'exception that proves the rule' and therefore has difficulty in answering an apparently simple question. This is a difficult dilemma, but in general it's probably best to ignore such personally-witnessed rarities unless you have seen them mentioned in standard textbooks.

Shortage of time is rarely a problem in M.C.Q. exams and therefore answers can be checked. In my experience however 'second thoughts' in M.C.Q. exams are rarely an improvement and I think it is preferable to work steadily through the paper once only, but noting any question which will require later thought.

The clinical examination

Examiners rightly lay great stress on 'the clinical' when assessing a candidate and adequate preparation for this part of the examination is vital. The major skill required is of course the ability to elicit physical signs correctly but other factors such as fluency in case presentation and clinical judgement in the interpretation of the signs elicited are also important. The best way to improve your style in 'the clinical' is to obtain regular coaching from a critical senior colleague who will point out your faults. Failing this, you should make arrangements with a fellow-student for each to see the other's cases under examination conditions. To obtain the maximum benefit you should of course 'grill' each other on the findings immediately afterwards. This method has the advantage that you will learn to see things from the examiner's point of view and you will quickly come to appreciate those bad habits which commonly cause annoyance to examiners.

Despite current trends, sartorial and tonsorial conservatism is recommended, as both patients and examiners are likely to be middle-aged if not actually senile. Attractive female candidates probably have an advantage but microskirts and low necklines may suggest that the girl who reveals all has something to hide.

The major ('long') case
History-taking

A successful history demands just as much skill as the physical examination, and while two experienced clinicians will usually agree on the physical signs the histories they obtain may be quite different. The examiners realize this and therefore attach more importance to the objective physical findings in assessing a candidate. An accurate history is important for diagnosis however, particularly with cardiological or neurological patients, who are frequently used as 'long' cases because of their stable physical signs. There is more to the assessment of a cardiological case than merely hearing and interpreting the murmurs, which, contrary to popular belief, are usually 'loud and clear' in examination cases. It is vitally important to obtain the fullest possible details of previous illnesses, especially with regard to the duration, symptoms and treatment of any possible bouts of rheumatic fever, chorea, tonsillitis, SABE, etc., and in female patients you must obtain full details of previous pregnancies. Male patients can often give the results of previous medical examinations performed for insurance purposes or for medical grading prior to service in the armed forces, and many patients can give the date and result of previous chest X-rays. Details of the patient's past and present exercise tolerance are of course essential, and you should ascertain from the patient exactly how much physical effort his present work entails. In neurology cases the mode of onset (over minutes, days or weeks), length of history and subsequent course (static, steadily progressive or remitting) will usually suggest the type of pathological lesion present (e.g. vascular, inflammatory, neoplastic or degenerative), and the physical signs will then confirm the anatomical site of the lesion.

When taking a history in exams it is advisable first to list all the patient's symptoms briefly, to discover the type of illness and the systems involved. The symptoms should then be arranged chronologically and full details about each should be obtained. Thus if the patient complains of pain you should determine:

1. The site, with the direction of radiation.
2. Its nature and severity.
3. Its duration and periodicity.
4. Any aggravating or relieving factors.
5. Any associated features.

Think about the possible diagnosis from the outset and modify your questions accordingly.

Never accept terms such as rheumatism and vertigo at their face value but ask the patient what he means by this. You may be surprised, as was the G.P. who gave several prescriptions for bigger and better laxatives for an old dear who was 'costive', until he discovered she thought this was a synonym for diarrhoea.

Considerable persistence may be needed to prevent the patient digressing. With garrulous patients the previous medical and family histories are particularly difficult to obtain. In such cases stick to essentials and don't hesitate to ask leading questions in order to obtain the necessary information.

The history will allow you to assess the patient's mood, intellect, speech and memory, and you should of course observe the patient closely during the history for signs of dyspnoea, tremor, etc. It is also a good idea on first meeting the patient to ask yourself 'Could this be myxoedema?' as this diagnosis is otherwise easily missed.

Examination

The ability to elicit and interpret physical signs is of course essential and considerable practise on the wards is required to achieve this skill. A combination of speed and thoroughness is required for exam purposes, and this applies especially to pulmonary percussion, cardiac auscultation and examination of the C.N.S. In auscultation in particular, first impressions are often right and prolonged listening may cause confusion. It's usually more convenient to examine a patient from the head downwards, rather than by systems, and regular practise with an unvarying routine is required if no major points are to be missed. I cannot stress too strongly that people fail their long case not through missing a minor abnormality, but because in their haste they have failed to look for a sign which is in fact present in a gross form. Obvious signs such as a large breast mass, hypertension, marked tracheal shift, gross optic atrophy, unilateral deafness, severe intention tremor, massive splenomegaly, etc., can easily be missed unless the appropriate examination is performed. Such signs may not always be suspected to be present from the history, although it is of course advisable to pay special attention to the systems where you expect positive findings. Thus it would be foolish to accept the absence of a mitral murmur too readily in a patient with dyspnoea, haemoptysis, and a malar flush, or to be satisfied with perfunctory palpation for splenomegaly in a patient with suspected leukaemia.

Equivocal findings can usually be safely ignored unless they are relevant to the symptoms or probable diagnosis. For example it is best not to waste much time over minor degrees of reflex inequality, slight facial asymmetry, impaired vibration sense, etc., unless your patient has a neurological disorder, or a disease which causes a neuropathy. Other common causes of real or imagined equivocation which can often be ignored include slight bilateral pallor or blurring of the optic disc, slight tracheal or apical displacement, soft murmurs and slight inequality of breath sounds. Remember that small differences in percussion are easily imagined and bronchial breathing is uncommon. If a finding is dubious and it doesn't fit, forget it.

For the major case practise working well within the set time-limit, so that you have time left at the end to recheck your positive findings and to look again for any associated signs which you might expect to be present in that particular case. Remember that mistakes in the history may occasionally be explained away as being due to the patient's poor memory, but mistakes in the physical signs are entirely the responsibility of the candidate and cannot be condoned.

On completion of the examination you should carefully consider the possible diagnoses and then clarify any doubtful points in the history. You should also amplify the history regarding any unexpected physical signs you have discovered.

Quite apart from any humanitarian considerations it is most important to try to establish a good rapport with your patient. Many of the patients used in the examination are chronic cases with more or less stable physical signs. Since such patients are in frequent demand for teaching purposes they usually have a long experience of young doctors and their difficulties and they are often well aware which of their own physical signs are commonly missed. Occasionally such patients will spontaneously volunteer valuable information with regard to their diagnosis or physical signs, but in other cases a judiciously worded question at the end of your examination such as 'Is there anything else you think I ought to know?' will often prove rewarding. Other useful clues may be obtained by asking the patient to describe the investigations and treatment he has had, and by asking him what he believes to be the cause of his symptoms. Occasionally you'll hit the jackpot with a reply such as 'Well the doctors at Queen Square said it was Frederick Attacks Yer'. You must be prepared for misleading answers however, and these should be ignored if they do not tally with your own assessment of the history and physical signs. These questions should be left until the end as otherwise the replies will prejudice your judgement. Another point to consider is that these questions sometimes provoke in the patient an uncooperative attitude of 'That's for me to know and you to find out' which can make subsequent history-taking difficult.

Before the examiner arrives you should reconsider your diagnosis and ask yourself 'Could this be anything else?' Remember that elderly patients often have multiple pathology, and remember too that although rare diseases occur rarely, their prevalence in examinations is greatly increased. If the diagnosis is uncertain prepare a list of differential diagnoses and consider what investigations you would perform, remembering to mention simple tests such as E.S.R. and chest radiograph before more expensive and possibly dangerous procedures. In most Final M.B. exams simple urine tests are required as part of the physical examination of the patient and this important step should not be forgotten. If there is time, you should consider how you would answer probable questions regarding management and prognosis, and in appropriate cases you should try to anticipate what the ECG and radiographs might show.

Case presentation

There is quite an art in presenting a case concisely and clearly. The examiners have no time to waste, and hesitant and long-winded presentations are tedious, so you should edit the history, emphasizing important points, leaving out irrelevant detail and giving negatives only if they are important. If the case is straightforward the presentation of the history and examination should form a cohesive account leading to a confident diagnosis. In such cases try to make your assessment as full as you can and say whether the condition in your patient is acute or chronic, mild or severe, simple or with complications. In more difficult cases with conflicting evidence or doubtful signs you will have more reservations, but don't hedge all the time as this irritates examiners and does nothing to conceal your ignorance. Try to make up your mind on the basis of probabilities. Doctors often have to act on the basis of equivocal evidence and the examiners want to see whether you can take a sensible decision.

While it is important to keep your initial presentation concise, it is a mistake to answer the subsequent questions too curtly. The examiner is anxious to see whether you can discuss your patient intelligently and you should try to display your relevant knowledge as much as possible. If anything about the case puzzles you, or there is a problem relating to diagnosis or management, don't be afraid to acknowledge this. If the line of questioning seems to be entering one of your fields of ignorance try to keep the initiative by talking around the subject. With a bit of luck you may introduce a fresh topic that interests the examiner. If he persists in reiterating a particular question this is often because he is trying to establish a very basic point. Examiners can be obtuse in the way they phrase such questions and prolonged silences in such circumstances can be disastrous. Try to talk sensibly around the subject to see what he's aiming at, and with luck a supplementary question will lead you to the required answer.

The minor ('short') cases

Many students regard the minor cases as a little light relief from the more arduous parts of the examination. This is a serious misconception, for the examiners are well aware of the element of luck which enters into the major case, and they attach correspondingly greater importance to the candidate's performance while he is under direct observation. You will be watched as you examine the patient and your style in eliciting physical signs is important. Make a point of positioning the patient properly, and although you should preserve the patient's modesty as far as possible, remember that you may be penalized if you do not get the patient adequately undressed.

As in the long cases, a reasonable compromise must be reached between speed and thoroughness in physical examination, for as a general rule a candidate's score is proportional to the number of cases he has time to examine and diagnose correctly. It is obviously better to err on the side of over-caution rather than to fail because of a major error of omission, but remember that few things irritate an examiner more than the candidate who wastes time performing a tediously meticulous examination in what should be a simple, rapidly diagnosed condition. The examination of the sensory nervous system often provides cause for offence in this respect, and cardiological auscultation presents a similar hazard. If you are unsure of the diagnosis in a case with an 'interesting' murmur, there is usually no point in remaining glued to the patient's praecordium in the hope of being saved by the bell, for the examiner will certainly ask you for a diagnosis before dismissing you. Far better to think quickly, present a sensible differential diagnosis and move on to the next case.

Another important point in the minor cases is to listen carefully to the instructions of the examiner with regard to the part or system to be examined and obey them implicitly. Before recounting your findings however you should always pause and ask yourself whether further examination of more distant parts of the body such as regional lymph nodes, peripheral pulses, finger nails, etc., is required.

The importance of the recognition of clinical associations in the minor cases cannot be overemphasized. In many cases inspection of the patient and his immediate environment as you approach the bed may provide a clue to the diagnosis. For example you may be shown a cutaneous eruption localized to the shin in a patient with exophthalmos (pretibial myxoedema), or you may be asked to give the likely diagnosis of an arthritis in a patient who also has a patch of psoriasis, or marked nail pitting. The key to many minor cases lies in such observations and you should practise looking for such clinical associations until this becomes habitual.

Having elicited the physical signs correctly many candidates fail to be selective enough in applying their knowledge to the particular patient under discussion. Blind application of 'lists of causes' oblivious of the patient's age or sex, the associated physical findings, etc., are guaranteed to create a poor impression. The habit of mentioning rare diseases before common ones is another failing which is easily eradicated with practice.

Hints and tips received from earlier candidates in the short cases are on the whole best ignored. Examiners have been known to change the order of the patients' beds and they will certainly have changed the questions. There is moreover a real danger that you will jump to the diagnosis (which may in any case be wrong) without giving adequate consideration to the differential diagnoses and without eliciting the appropriate physical signs.

It is heartening to realize that for success in the clinical examination omniscience helps, but is by no means essential (indeed a few examiners seem to find it somewhat irritating). More important are adequate practise in examination technique, quick-wittedness, thoroughness, clear enunciation, a confident but modest bearing, and good luck.

The oral examination ('viva')

The 'viva' tests the depth as well as the breadth of a candidate's knowledge. If he appears to know a topic fairly well the examiners will switch to another subject and if several common topics are satisfactorily dealt with they may go on to test the candidate 'in depth'. For this reason it may be worthwhile for the good candidate to learn about a few unusual multisystem conditions in detail and to try and introduce them into the conversation. For example a student who has spent an elective period in the U.S.A. might choose coccidioidomycosis as a subject to revise in detail. Then if he is asked about pneumonia, meningitis, osteomyelitis, tuberculosis, erythema nodosum or lymphadenopathy he will, after discussing the commoner causes, casually mention coccidioidomycosis. The examiner will often rise to the bait and say 'Ah yes, now what do you know about that?'

The converse of this ploy is that you should not mention anything in the 'viva' unless you're prepared to talk about it. For the same reason you should avoid the use of words such as atelectasis and rales, whose definition is controversial, unless you can discuss the terminology in detail.

You may be given a pathology specimen ('pot') to describe in the viva. Examine it carefully from all sides to try to identify the organ first (not always easy), then describe the pathological lesions you can see, and hazard a diagnosis. If you know the answer try to talk at some length. If you haven't a clue, don't prevaricate but have a guess and go on to the next 'pot'. Tipping it upside down to look at the label is not recommended as it will only make the 'pot' too cloudy to see anything!

If you are shown a radiograph the abnormality is likely to be fairly gross so stand back and take an overall view before looking at the details. Remember that more than one abnormality may be present (e.g. an absent breast shadow with pulmonary metastases, or a bronchial cancer with rib metastases) so examine the whole film. Assuming you can spot the abnormality it is best to discuss this from the outset as examiners get tired of being told that the patient is slightly rotated and the film is of poor quality.

Finally, have sympathy with your examiner. He cannot be expected to know everything and if you cross swords with him, give ground gracefully—after all he may be right!

Cardiology

CYANOSIS

5 gm reduced Hb per 100 ml blood produces cyanosis

PERIPHERAL CYANOSIS

Due to poor peripheral circulation

Causes

1. Cardiac failure
2. Vasoconstriction
3. Arterial obstruction

CENTRAL CYANOSIS

Due to inadequate oxygenation

Causes

1. Decreased pO_2 of inspired gas
2. Hypoventilation
3. Lung disease
4. R to L cardiac shunt

May be simulated by methaemoglobinaemia and sulphaemoglobinaemia

JUGULAR VENOUS PULSE

Height of JVP is measured with reference to sternal angle with subject at 30° to horizontal
Normally less than 4 cm (vertical height)

Causes of elevated JVP

1. Hyperdynamic circulation:
    (i)   Exercise
    (ii) Fever
    (iii) Anaemia
    (iv) Thyrotoxicosis
    (v)   Pregnancy
    (vi) AV fistulae

2. R ventricular failure
3. Obstruction of superior vena cava
4. Tricuspid stenosis or incompetence
5. Pericardial effusion or constrictive pericarditis
6. Fluid overload (esp. IV infusion)
7. Very slow heart rate

TYPES OF ARTERIAL PULSE WAVE

1. **Normal**

2. **Collapsing**
   (i)   Aortic incompetence
   (ii) Hyperdynamic circulation
   (iii) Patent ductus arteriosus
   (iv) Peripheral AV aneurysms
   (v)   Arteriosclerotic aorta

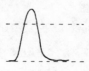

3. **Plateau**
   Aortic stenosis

4. **Small volume**
   (i)   'Shock'
   (ii) Aortic stenosis
   (iii) Pericardial effusion

5. **Bisferiens**
   Combined aortic stenosis
   and incompetence

6. **Anacrotic**
   Aortic stenosis

7. **Dicrotic**
   Fevers

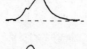

8. **Pulsus alternans**—Alternate strong and weak beats
   Left ventricular failure
9. **Pulsus paradoxus**—Volume decreases on inspiration
   (i)   Pericardial effusion
   (ii) Constrictive pericarditis

CLINICAL DIAGNOSIS OF AN ARRHYTHMIA

1. **Sinus arrhythmia**—rate increases with inspiration

2. **Extrasystoles** Atrial, nodal or ventricular
   - (i)   a premature beat with a compensatory pause followed by a stronger beat
   - (ii) usually runs of normal beats occur, but extrasystoles may alternate with normal beats (pulsus bigeminus)
   - (iii) may disappear during exercise

3. **Atrial fibrillation**
   - (i)   completely irregular in time and force
   - (ii) worse on exercise
   - (iii) carotid compression has no effect
   - (iv) JVP 'a' waves absent

4. **Atrial flutter**
   - (i)   regular radial pulse rate 125–160/min
   - (ii) AV block occurs, so that the JVP 'a' waves greatly exceed the pulse rate
   - (iii) carotid compression slows the rate while pressure is maintained

5. **Paroxysmal tachycardia** Atrial, nodal or ventricular
   - (i)   may be history of previous attacks with sudden onset and cessation
   - (ii) carotid compression may decrease the rate even after pressure is relaxed

6. **Heart block**

Complete (3rd degree)—	Heart rate of 36–44/min which does not increase with exercise
2nd degree AV block—	May be dropped beats (Wenckebach) or 2:1, 3:1 or 4:1 block Instability of rhythm is common.
1st degree block—	Difficult to identify clinically, (PR>0·2 second on ECG)

COMMON CAUSES OF SOME ARRHYTHMIAS

Extrasystoles
1. Idiopathic
2. Fatigue, excessive smoking, alcohol or caffeine ingestion
3. Myocardial ischaemia
4. Digitalis
5. Hyperthyroidism
6. Heart diseases with atrial enlargement (e.g. mitral stenosis)

Paroxysmal tachycardia
1. Myocardial ischaemia
2. Digitalis, especially after potassium depletion
3. Cor pulmonale

Atrial fibrillation
1. Rh. heart disease, especially mitral stenosis
2. Myocardial ischaemia
3. Hyperthyroidism

Heart block (all degrees)
1. Myocardial ischaemia
2. Digitalis
3. Chronic heart disease, especially aortic stenosis and congenital lesions
4. Acute infectious disease, including rheumatic fever

APEX BEAT

Heart is enlarged or displaced if apex beat is:

   (i) lateral to midclavicular line, or
   (ii) below 5th intercostal space

Tapping apex beat indicates RV hypertrophy, but a left parasternal heave is more reliable

Causes of absent apex beat
   (1) Obesity
   (2) Emphysema
   (3) Pericardial effusion
   (4) Shock
   (5) Dextrocardia

Remember that apex beat in axillary line is often missed

THRILLS
Always indicate an organic defect
The area localizes the defect

Important causes
Systolic
1. At apex (i) Ventricular septal defect
       (ii) Mitral incompetence (rarely)
2. At base on right (i) Aortic stenosis
              (ii) Aortic aneurysm
3. At base on left—Congenital heart disease, esp. pulmonary stenosis

Diastolic
1. At apex—Mitral stenosis
2. At base—Aortic incompetence.

LEFT VENTRICULAR FAILURE
Common causes
1. Myocardial ischaemia
2. Hypertension
3. Aortic stenosis or incompetence
4. Mitral incompetence

Symptoms
1. Exertional dyspnoea
2. Orthopnoea
3. Paroxysmal nocturnal dyspnoea, often with coughing or wheezing
4. Pulmonary oedema (anxiety, dyspnoea, cough and pink frothy sputum)

Signs
1. Tachycardia. May be pulsus alternans
2. Enlarged heart
3. Gallop rhythm
4. May be functional mitral incompetence due to stretched AV ring
5. Crepitations at lung bases
May be rhonchi
6. Cheyne-Stokes respirations may occur in sedated elderly patients

RIGHT VENTRICULAR FAILURE
Common causes
1. Secondary to L ventricular failure
2. Mitral stenosis
3. Cor pulmonale (including pulmonary embolism)
4. Congenital heart disease

Symptoms
1. Tiredness, weakness, anorexia
2. Oedema
3. Gastro-intestinal upset. May be hepatic pain

Signs
1. Dependent oedema
2. Elevated JVP
3. May be functional tricuspid incompetence due to stretched AV ring
4. Large tender liver. May be mild jaundice
5. May be ascites or pleural effusion
6. Oliguria by day and nocturia. Urine is concentrated and albuminuria is common
7. Peripheral cyanosis in severe cases

Remember that R and L sided heart failure often appear almost simultaneously

CAUSES OF SYSTEMIC HYPERTENSION
1. Essential
2. Renal disease (especially renal ischaemia)
3. Cushing's disease or glucocorticoid therapy
4. Phaeochromocytoma
5. Primary aldosteronism (Conn's)
6. Coarctation (but B.P. normal in legs)
7. Toxaemia of pregnancy

HEART SOUNDS

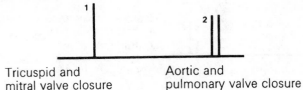

Tricuspid and
mitral valve closure

Aortic and
pulmonary valve closure

N.B.
1. Aortic normally closes before pulmonary
2. Pulmonary closure is delayed by inspiration (due to
   increased venous return caused by decreased intrathoracic
   pressure)
The normal split therefore widens on inspiration

First sound

Loud in
   1. mitral stenosis
   2. hyperdynamic circulation
   3. tachycardia
Soft in
   1. mitral incompetence
   2. rheumatic carditis
   3. severe heart failure

Second sound in aortic area

Loud in systemic hypertension
Soft in aortic stenosis

Second sound in pulmonary area

Loud in pulmonary hypertension
Soft in pulmonary stenosis

Third heart sound

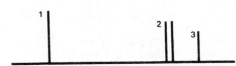

Heard at apex early in
diastole, due to ventricular
distension
Easily confused with
opening snap of mitral
stenosis which is maximal
medial to the apex

Causes:
   (i)   Normal in young people (but abnormal after 40)
   (ii) Ventricular failure
   (iii) Constrictive pericarditis
   (iv) Mitral or tricuspid incompetence

(continued)

Fourth heart sound

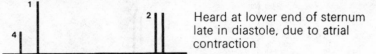

Heard at lower end of sternum late in diastole, due to atrial contraction

Always abnormal, indicates resistance to LV filling

Causes:

(i) Hypertension
(ii) Heart block

Triple rhythm is due to a 3rd or 4th heart sound, or summation of both
Gallop rhythm is a fast triple rhythm, and indicates actual or incipient heart failure
Dogmatic pronouncements on the state of the second sound and the presence or absence of the third and fourth sounds are not normally expected of undergraduates

CARDIAC MURMURS

When auscultating, concentrate separately on the heart rhythm, sounds and murmurs. The murmurs most commonly missed in exams are those of aortic incompetence and mitral stenosis. Aortic incompetence is missed either because auscultation was not performed all down the L sternal edge with the patient sitting up at the end of expiration, or because the candidate failed to 'tune-in' to the high-pitched murmur. Mitral stenosis is missed either because the patient was not auscultated lying on his left side, or because the candidate listened to only one site in the apical area. A loud first heart sound should suggest the possibility of a mitral stenosis murmur. If several murmurs are present, try to decide which lesion is dominant by consideration of associated clinical features, e.g. in simultaneous AS and AI the pulse may be either 'plateau' or 'collapsing', and in simultaneous MS and MI the presence of a 3rd heart sound with a soft 1st sound suggests the incompetence is dominant.

If no murmur is heard and the patient gives a history of rheumatic fever, you should exercise the patient and listen again.

In any patient in whom you suspect rheumatic heart disease you should obtain details of the symptoms, duration and treatment of any previous bouts of possible rheumatic fever, chorea, tonsillitis or bacterial endocarditis.

MITRAL STENOSIS

Nearly always due to rheumatic heart disease, but rarely may be congenital

Symptoms

1. Progressive exertional dyspnoea
2. Other symptoms of pulmonary congestion:
    Orthopnoea
    Paroxysmal nocturnal dyspnoea
    Cough
    Haemoptysis
3. Acute pulmonary oedema, usually precipitated by exertion or pregnancy
4. Recurrent bronchitis
5. In later stages, symptoms of RV failure (p. 16)

Signs

1. Thin face with purple cheeks ('mitral facies')
2. Pulse may be small volume. May be atrial fibrillation
3. B.P. shows low pulse pressure
4. May be 'tapping' apex beat and L parasternal heave
    May be diastolic thrill
5. 1st heart sound is loud and 'slapping'
    2nd heart sound is loud if pulmonary hypertension is present
    May be 'opening snap' (indicates mobile valve)
6. Rough, rumbling low-pitched diastolic murmur, localized to the apical area and accentuated by exercise. May be presystolic crescendo if fibrillation absent. Severity of stenosis is indicated by *duration* not loudness of murmur
7. Pulmonary crepitations
8. In later stages, signs of RV failure (p. 16)

Complications

1. Thrombi in L atrium, and systemic embolization
2. Venous thrombosis and pulmonary emboli
3. Subacute bacterial endocarditis (uncommon with atrial fibrillation)

Electrocardiogram

1. May be broad notched P wave
2. May be atrial fibrillation
3. R axis deviation or R ventricular hypertrophy
4. Usually digitalis effects

MITRAL INCOMPETENCE
Symptoms
1. Palpitations and exertional dyspnoea occur early
2. Fatigue and weakness
3. Pulmonary oedema

Signs
1. L ventricular hypertrophy
2. 1st heart sound is soft and muffled
   3rd heart sound is usual
3. Loud pansystolic murmur, maximal at apex and propagated to axilla
   Often obscures 2nd heart sound
4. May be LV failure

AORTIC STENOSIS
Symptoms
1. May be none for years
2. Symptoms of L ventricular failure (p. 15)
3. Syncope or angina on effort

Signs
1. Small volume 'plateau' pulse
2. L ventricular hypertrophy
   May be systolic thrill (best felt with patient sitting forward at end of expiration)
3. 2nd sound in aortic area is soft
4. Harsh systolic 'ejection' murmur maximal at aortic area and propagated to the neck
5. May be LV failure

Aortic sclerosis murmur is identical, but is distinguished by normal radial pulse wave and absence of a thrill

AORTIC INCOMPETENCE
Symptoms
1. May be none for many years
2. Palpitations and dizziness
3. Symptoms of L ventricular failure (p. 15)
4. Angina

Signs
1. Collapsing (Corrigan) pulse
   May be visible carotid pulsation or 'head-nodding' or nail bed pulsation
2. B.P. shows wide pulse pressure
3. L ventricular hypertrophy
4. Murmurs:

    (i) Soft high-pitched blowing diastolic murmur down L sternal edge
    (ii) May be a systolic aortic murmur due to increased blood flow
    (iii) May be a diastolic apical murmur (Austin Flint) which simulates mitral stenosis
    (iv) May be 'pistol-shot' noise over femorals synchronous with pulse
    (v) May be diastolic murmur over femorals on slight compression with stethoscope bell

5. May be LV failure

TRICUSPID INCOMPETENCE

Clinical manifestations usually determined by coexisting and predominating mitral stenosis

Symptoms
1. Exertional dyspnoea is common, but orthopnoea and paroxysmal nocturnal dyspnoea are uncommon due to diminished R ventricular output into lungs
2. Gastro-intestinal upsets due to venous congestion of GI tract

Signs
1. Elevated JVP with large v waves
2. Pulsatile hepatic enlargement
3. Ascites, which is both chronic and recurrent
4. Peripheral oedema, pleural effusions
5. Pansystolic murmur, maximal near lower sternum, and becoming louder during deep inspiration

CLASSIFICATION OF CONGENITAL HEART DISEASES

(A) **Cyanotic** (i.e. R to L shunt)

- (i) Fallot's tetrad :
    pulmonary stenosis
    ventricular septal defect
    over-riding aorta
    right ventricular hypertrophy
- (ii) Eisenmenger complex (VSD with pulmonary hypertension)
- (iii) Transposition of great vessels and tricuspid atresia are usually fatal in infancy

(B) **Acyanotic**

(1) With L to R shunt

- (i) Ventricular septal defect
- (ii) Atrial septal defect—usually secundum but rarely septum primum
- (iii) Persistent ductus arteriosus

These patients may become cyanosed due to cardiac failure, pulmonary infection or severe exercise

(2) With no shunt

- (i) Coarctation of aorta
- (ii) Pulmonary stenosis—occasionally cyanosed
- (iii) Congenital aortic stenosis
- (iv) Dextrocardia
- (v) Bicuspid aortic valves

DIFFERENTIAL DIAGNOSIS OF MURMURS

Timing	Maximal intensity	Likely causes
Ejection systolic	Aortic area	Aortic stenosis Aortic sclerosis Aortic aneurysm Coarctation
	Pulmonary area	Innocent Pulmonary stenosis Atrial septal defect Pulmonary hypertension
	Apex	Innocent Aortic stenosis Aortic sclerosis
Pansystolic	Apex	Mitral incompetence (functional or organic) Ventricular septal defect Fallot's tetrad
	Lower sternal border	Tricuspid incompetence (functional or organic)
Diastolic	Apex	Mitral stenosis
	Lower sternal border	Tricuspid stenosis
	Anywhere along sternal border	Aortic incompetence Pulmonary incompetence Bacterial endocarditis
Continuous ('To and fro')	Cardiac base	Patent ductus arteriosus Simultaneous AS and AI
	Above clavicle	Venous 'hum'

Remember the possibility of extracardiac sounds such as pericarditis

Causes of severe chest pain

1. Myocardial ischaemia

    (i)   coronary atheroma, thrombus or vasospasm
    (ii) aortic valve disease or aortitis
    (iii) severe anaemia
    (iv) paroxysmal tachycardia

2. Pericarditis
3. Pleurisy or pneumothorax
4. Pulmonary embolism
5. Oesophageal pain (acid reflux, spasm, carcinoma)
6. Chest wall lesions

    (i)   rib fracture
    (ii) metastatic deposits in ribs
    (iii) fibrositis or myalgia
    (iv) herpes zoster

7. Gastric or duodenal ulcer
8. Gallbladder colic
9. Pain referred from thoracic or cervical spine
10. Aortic aneurysm

Complications of myocardial infarction

1. Cardiac arrhythmia
    (i)   Sinus or nodal bradycardia
    (ii) Supraventricular tachycardia, atrial flutter, atrial fibrillation
    (iii) Ventricular tachycardia, flutter or fibrillation
    (iv) Heart block
    (v)   Cardiac asystole
2. Left ventricular failure
3. Hypotension
4. 'Shock'
5. Pulmonary embolism (usually from leg veins)
6. Mural thrombus and systemic emboli
7. Pericarditis
8. Ruptured papillary muscle or chordae tendineae
9. Ventricular septal defect
10. Cardiac aneurysm or rupture
11. Dressler's syndrome
12. Psychological, including 'L. chest pain'
13. Frozen shoulder and 'shoulder hand' syndrome
14. Iatrogenic; drugs, pacing, etc.

COR PULMONALE

Cardiac disease secondary to chronic disease of lungs or pulmonary vessels

Causes

1. Emphysema and chronic bronchitis
2. Pulmonary fibrosis
3. Multiple pulmonary emboli
4. Severe kyphoscoliosis

Signs of cor pulmonale

1. Warm cyanosed extremities with bounding pulse
2. Raised JVP, hepatomegaly and oedema
3. Triple rhythm and loud P2 due to pulmonary hypertension (but overlying emphysema may cause soft heart sounds)
4. Functional tricuspid incompetence in severe cases

PERICARDITIS

Causes

1. Myocardial infarct
2. Benign (usually viral)
3. Rheumatic fever
4. Pyogenic (pneumonia or septicaemia)
5. Tuberculous
6. Cancer invading the pericardium (bronchus or breast)
7. Severe uraemia
8. SLE

RAYNAUD'S PHENOMENON

Causes

1. *Reflex vasoconstriction*

    (i) Raynaud's disease
    (ii) Vibrating machinery

2. *Arterial occlusion*

    (i) Thoracic outlet syndromes
    (ii) Atheroma, Buerger's disease

3. *Collagen-vascular disease,* especially systemic sclerosis
4. *Increased blood viscosity*

    (i) Dysproteinaemias (macro- and cryo-globulinaemias)
    (ii) Polycythaemia, leukaemia

5. *Neurological disease,* especially syringomyelia or paralysis

Electrocardiography

THE NORMAL ELECTROCARDIOGRAM

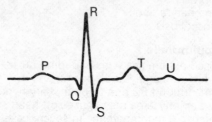

PR should be < 0·20 sec
QRS should be < 0·12 sec
1 large square (5 mm) on ECG paper = 0·2 sec

∴ Ventricular rate/minute = $\dfrac{300}{\text{No. of large squares between adjacent R peaks}}$

Standard leads

ECG interpretation is facilitated by imagining that the standard leads 'look at' the electrical activity of the heart from the following viewpoints in a coronal plane:

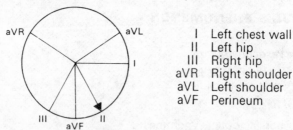

I	Left chest wall
II	Left hip
III	Right hip
aVR	Right shoulder
aVL	Left shoulder
aVF	Perineum

The greatest positive deflection (R wave, due to left ventricular depolarization) is thus normally seen in lead II, and this is the *'cardiac axis'* (see arrow). Right or left axis deviation is thus detected by examining R in the standard leads

Chest leads

These leads 'look at' the heart in a horizontal plane from the right of the sternum (VI) to the axillary line (V6)

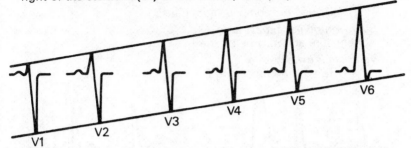

Clockwise or anti-clockwise rotation is thus detected by these leads

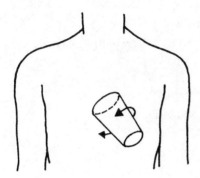

ARRHYTHMIAS

1. Premature beats

Arise from ectopic focus in atrium, AV node or ventricle
Usually followed by 'compensatory pause'

Supraventricular extrasystole
P is premature and may be bizarre

Ventricular extrasystole
Bizarre QRS with no preceding P

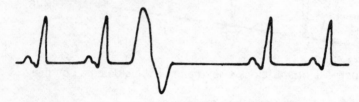

2. Paroxysmal atrial tachycardia

Normal QRS, but T waves altered by fusion with P waves

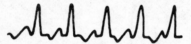

PAT with block (usually induced by digitalis)
Rapid regular P waves with slower QRS waves

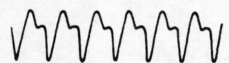

3. Paroxysmal ventricular tachycardia

QRS complexes are slurred and wide but fairly regular
P waves often obscured

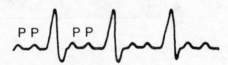

4. Atrial fibrillation

Absent P waves and QRS complexes completely irregular

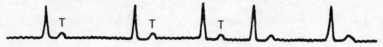

VENTRICULAR HYPERTROPHY

LVH

1. Tall R waves in left chest leads with deep S waves in right chest leads
   Sum of S in VI and R in V5 exceeds 37 mm
2. May be LV 'strain' (ST depression and T inversion)
3. Left axis deviation
4. QRS may be slightly prolonged

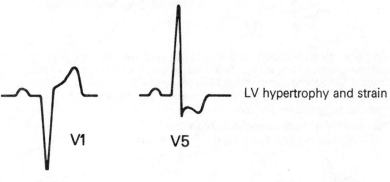

V1   V5   LV hypertrophy and strain

RVH

1. Tall R waves in right chest leads with S waves in left chest leads
2. R axis deviation

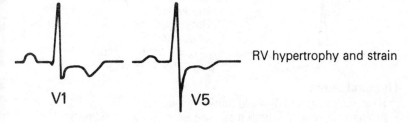

V1   V5   RV hypertrophy and strain

Myocardial infarction

Characteristic changes are:
1. Appearance of Q waves exceeding 0·04 sec
2. ST elevation and T wave inversion in leads facing the infarct
3. ST depression in leads diametrically opposite the infarct

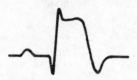

Recent myocardial infarct

Anterior infarct—usually due to occlusion of the descending L coronary artery. The infarct faces leads I, aVL and the chest leads
Inferior (diaphragmatic) infarct—faces leads II, III and aVF
Persistence of the acute infarction pattern for more than 6 months suggests ventricular aneurysm

Myocardial ischaemia without infarction

ST depression and symmetrical T wave inversion

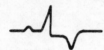

Digitalis also causes ST depression and T inversion but in a 'reversed tick' pattern

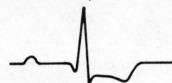

Digitalis also causes:
1. Bradycardia
2. Prolonged PR
3. Shortened QT
4. Any arrhythmia, especially bigemini or heart block

Hypokalaemia

ST depression and T wave flattening or inversion
Prominent U waves, which may fuse with the succeeding P

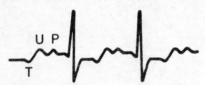

Hyperkalaemia

Small P waves with tall peaked T waves
QRS complex widens, and ventricular fibrillation may follow

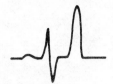

Pericarditis

(i) *Acute* ST elevation in all the standard leads except aVR, and in most of the chest leads

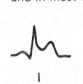   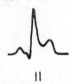   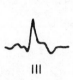

I   II   III

(ii) *Chronic* ST becomes isoelectric and the T wave flattens and may invert

Acute pulmonary embolism

1. T wave inversion and Q wave in leads III and VI—V3
2. Transient RBBB
3. Right axis deviation

Cor pulmonale

1. Large pointed P waves
2. Changes of RV hypertrophy

Chest disease

LUNG VOLUMES

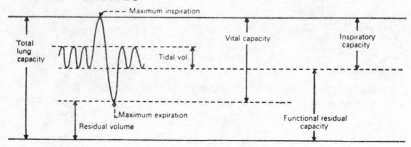

The resting expiratory level is the most constant reference point on the spirometer tracing

Minute ventilation—product of tidal volume and number of respirations per minute

Vital capacity—largest volume a subject can expire after a single maximal inspiration. Normal values increase with size of subject and decrease with age (about $4\frac{1}{2}$ litres in young adult male). Can be reduced in practically any lung or chest wall disease

Forced vital capacity (FVC)—the vital capacity when the expiration is performed as rapidly as possible

FEV₁ (Forced expiratory volume in one second)—volume expired during first second of FVC

Ratio $\dfrac{FEV_1}{FVC}$ should be 75 per cent or more, and is reduced in obstructive airway diseases (asthma, emphysema, bronchitis)

Peak flow—maximum expiratory flow rate achieved during a forced expiration. A convenient way to detect a reduction in ventilatory function. Also useful for serial measurements in the same patient and for assessing response to bronchial antispasmodics

Residual volume—obtained by subtracting expiratory reserve volume from functional residual capacity. Residual volume is normally 20 to 25 per cent of total lung capacity but increases in elderly, and in over-inflation of the lungs (emphysema, asthma)

Anatomical dead space—The volume of air in the mouth, pharynx, trachea and bronchi up to the terminal bronchioles (about 150 ml). In disease the physiological dead space may greatly exceed the anatomical dead space due to disorders of the ventilation/perfusion ratio, but in health the two are identical

DIFFUSION DEFECTS

Carbon dioxide is about 20 times more diffusible than oxygen. In diffusion defects the *arterial pO_2* is normal or slightly reduced at rest, but decreases markedly after exercise due to increased tissue uptake of O_2. *Arterial pCO_2* is normal or even reduced at rest (due to hyperventilation) and tends to fall on exercise

Causes of reduced diffusing capacity

1. Alveolo-capillary block

    (i)   pulmonary oedema
    (ii) pulmonary fibrosis
    (iii) infiltrative lesions, e.g. sarcoidosis and lymphangitis
          carcinomatosa

2. Reduction in area available for diffusion

    (i) emphysema
    (ii) multiple pulmonary emboli

Lung compliance

A measure of lung elasticity. Compliance is reduced when the lungs are abnormally stiff due to pulmonary venous congestion or infiltrative or fibrotic lesions of the lungs

BLOOD-GAS ANALYSIS

These values must be related to the normal levels expected for the subject, e.g. baby, old man, pregnant woman

Hypoxia is oxygen deficiency at a specified site

Hypoxaemia is oxygen deficiency in the blood
In arterial blood of normal resting adult,

pCO_2 is about 40 mm Hg
pO_2 is about 80 to 100 mm Hg

Causes of hypoxaemia
1. Cardio-respiratory disorders
    (i)   Hypoventilation
    (ii) Abnormality of ventilation/perfusion ratio
    (iii) Impaired diffusion
    (iv) Venous to arterial shunt
2. Decreased pO_2 of inspired gas, e.g. high altitude
3. Reduction in active haemoglobin, e.g. coal gas poisoning

Dyspnoea is a subjective awareness of the need for an increased respiratory effort

Hypoventilation is a reduction in lung ventilation sufficient to cause hypercapnia

Kussmaul's breathing (air hunger). Occurs in acidosis (uraemia, diabetes mellitus) due to stimulation of respiratory centre

Cheyne–Stokes breathing—amplitude of respiration progressively deepens to a maximum, then decreases to a period of apnoea. Due to diminished sensitivity of respiratory centre to CO_2. Occurs in left ventricular failure, central respiratory depression and in normal infants

Oxygen therapy

In chronic hypoxia due to hypoventilation (e.g. chronic bronchitis, asthma), the arterial pCO_2 is raised and correction of the hypoxia by oxygen in high concentration may release the respiratory centre from its 'anoxic drive' and produce CO_2 narcosis. Low-concentration oxygen masks such as the Ventimask or Edinburgh mask should be used, with serial blood gas analyses

In hypoxia due to impaired gas exchange (e.g. pneumonia, pulmonary oedema) high concentration masks such as the Polymask are required

Common causes of haemoptysis

Exclude spurious haemoptysis (nasal bleeding, etc.)

Respiratory
1. Bronchial carcinoma
2. Pulmonary tuberculosis
3. Bronchitis
4. Bronchiectasis
5. Lung abscess

Cardiovascular
1. Pulmonary infarct
2. Mitral stenosis
3. Acute left ventricular failure

Less common causes include:
1. Pneumonia, especially pneumococcal
2. Collagen-vascular disease, especially polyarteritis nodosa
3. Idiopathic pulmonary haemosiderosis
4. Bleeding diathesis
5. Mycoses
6. Foreign body

In many patients with a small haemoptysis and negative physical findings no cause is ever found despite follow-up with serial chest X Rays

PHYSICAL SIGNS IN LUNG DISEASE

	Chest wall movement	Mediastinum and trachea	Tactile vocal fremitus	Percussion note	Breath sounds	Added sounds
Large pleural effusion	Decreased on affected side	Shift to opposite side	Absent	Stony dull	Absent. May be bronchial (±whispering pectoriloquy) above fluid level	Absent. May be pleural rub above fluid
Consolidation	Decreased on affected side	Central	Increased	Dull	Bronchial	Fine or medium crepitations
Massive collapse	Decreased on affected side	Shift to affected side	Absent	Dull	Decreased	Absent
Fibrosis	Local flattening with decreased movement	Shift to affected side	Increased	Dull	Bronchial	May be coarse crepitations
Large pneumothorax	Decreased on affected side	Shift to opposite side	Decreased	Increased	Decreased	Absent unless bowel sounds are transmitted
Emphysema	Decreased bilaterally ('Barrel chest')	Central (except in unilateral emphysema)	Decreased	Increased	Decreased	Absent
Bronchitis	Decreased bilaterally ('Barrel chest')	Central	Normal or decreased	Increased	Decreased	Rhonchi and crepitations

Common causes of clubbing

Respiratory
1. Bronchial carcinoma
2. Chronic pulmonary suppuration

Cardiovascular
1. Bacterial endocarditis
2. Cyanotic congenital heart disease

Less common causes include:
1. Asbestosis, especially with mesothelioma
2. Fibrosing alveolitis
3. Ulcerative colitis
4. Crohn's disease
5. Cirrhosis
6..Thyrotoxicosis
7. Brachial arteriovenous aneurysm (unilateral)
8. Familial

Causes of pulmonary collapse

1. *Absorption collapse* (due to complete bronchial obstruction)
   (i) Intraluminal, e.g. foreign body, mucus or clot
   (ii) Mural, e.g. bronchial carcinoma or adenoma
   (iii) Extramural, e.g. peribronchial lymphadenopathy or aortic aneurysm
2. *Pneumothorax or pleural effusion*
   Remember that in absorption collapse the mediastinum shifts to the affected side, but in collapse due to air or fluid in the pleural space the mediastinum may shift to the opposite side

Causes of pleural effusion

(A) *Transudate* (less than 2 g protein/100 ml fluid)

1. Cardiac failure
2. Nephrotic syndrome
3. Hepatic failure

(B) *Exudate* (more than 2 g protein/100 ml fluid)

1. Pneumonia
2. Malignancy (bronchial Ca, secondary Ca, Hodgkin's or mesothelioma)
3. TB
4. Pulmonary infarction
5. Collagen-vascular disease (especially SLE)
6. Subphrenic abscess

Causes of pneumothorax

1. Traumatic
2. Iatrogenic, e.g. thoracentesis or surgery
3. Spontaneous

  (i) Subpleural bulla
  (ii) Emphysema
  (iii) Asthma
  (iv) TB
  (v) Lung abscess
  (vi) Pneumoconiosis

Causes of empyema

1. Pneumonia, especially lobar, or secondary to bronchial Ca
2. Lung abscess
3. Subphrenic abscess
4. Mediastinal sepsis
5. Chest wound or surgery
6. TB

Causes of acute pulmonary oedema

1. *Left heart failure*
     Atrial, e.g. mitral stenosis
     Ventricular, e.g. hypertension or myocardial infarct
2. *Overload of IV fluid*
3. *Inhalation of irritant gas,* e.g. chlorine
4. *Fulminating viral or bacterial pneumonia*
5. *Fat emboli*
6. *Neurogenic* (rare)
     Head injury or cerebro-vascular accident

BRONCHIECTASIS

Dilatation of the bronchi, usually accompanied by recurrent bronchial suppuration

Pathogenesis

Increased outward traction on the bronchi and weakness of the bronchial wall due to inflammation are both important

Causes

1. *Infection*
   - (i)   Bronchiolitis of infancy
   - (ii) Measles or pertussis in children
   - (iii) Post broncho-pneumonic collapse in adults
   - (iv) Commonly in post-primary TB, but apical, therefore secondary infection is unusual

2. *Bronchial stenosis or occlusion*
   - (i)   Adenoma or carcinoma
   - (ii) Foreign body or asthma casts
   - (iii) Lymphadenopathy

3. Pulmonary aspergillosis
4. Mucoviscidosis
5. Congenital
   e.g. associated with situs inversus (Kartagener's syndrome)
6. Many cases are idiopathic

Clinical features

1. Classical symptom—Cough with copious purulent sputum, especially on changing posture
2. Classical sign—Localized persistent coarse crepitations
3. May be asymptomatic
4. Malaise, intermittent fever, halitosis
5. Weight loss or 'failure to thrive'
6. Dyspnoea, cyanosis or clubbing
7. Haemoptysis ('dry bronchiectasis')
8. Signs of collapse or fibrosis
9. Coexisting chronic sinusitis is common

Complications

1. Recurrent pneumonia after upper respiratory infection
2. Recurrent dry pleurisy
3. Massive haemoptysis
4. Lung abscess, empyema or cerebral abscess
5. Cor pulmonale
6. Amyloidosis

PNEUMONIA
Anatomical classification
1. *Lobar*
   Due to virulent organisms such as 'epidemic' pneumococcus
   (e.g. Type 3) staphylococcus aureus or Friedlander's (Klebsiella)
2. *Segmental* ('Benign aspiration pneumonia')
   Due to organisms of low virulence
Often follows upper respiratory tract infections
3. *Lobular* ('Bronchopneumonia' if bilateral)
   Occurs in babies and elderly or debilitated patients
   Due to haemophilus influenzae, 'carrier' pneumococci,
   streptococci, TB

Aetiological classification
1. *Infective*

   (i) *Bacterial* See above
   Pneumonia may also be a feature of generalized bacterial
infections, e.g. brucellosis, typhoid fever, plague
   (ii) *Viral*
                Ornithosis
                Respiratory syncytial
                Influenza (usually secondary bacterial infection)
                Mumps (usually secondary bacterial infection)
                Cytomegalovirus
                URT viruses (adenovirus, rhinovirus, parainfluenza)
   (iii) *Rickettsial:* Typhus
                         Q fever
   (iv) *Mycoplasmal:* M. pneumoniae (Eaton agent)
   (v) *Yeasts and fungi*
                Candida
                Actinomyces
                Histoplasma
   (vi) *Protozoa and parasites*
                Toxoplasma
                Amoebae
                Pheumocystis carinii

2. *Allergic*
   Collagen-vascular disease (esp. polyarteritis nodosa)
   Stevens-Johnson syndrome (Erythema multiforme)

3. *Chemical agents*
   (i) Irritant gases: NH_3, SO_2, Cl, oxides of nitrogen
   (ii) Irritant liquids: Vomitus
                         Lipoid pneumonia

4. *Physical agents*—Irradiation

In discussing causes of pneumonia remember the possibility of
1. Pre-existing lung disease, e.g. bronchial carcinoma
                                    bronchiectasis
2. Inhalation pneumonia

    (i)   Oral and pharyngeal sepsis and sinusitis
    (ii) Oesophageal obstruction and pharyngeal pouch
    (iii) Alcoholic debauch, drowning or anaesthesia
    (iv) Laryngeal cancer
    (v) Tracheo-oesophageal fistula

3. Predisposing systemic disease such as diabetes, cirrhosis or agranulocytosis
4. Foreign body not seen on X-ray (e.g. peanut)

Complications of pneumococcal lobar pneumonia

1. Pleurisy with effusion, or serous pericarditis
2. Empyema or pericardial suppuration
3. Endocarditis, septicaemia, meningitis (not to be confused with meningismus, in which csf is normal) or cerebral abscess
4. Delayed resolution
5. Nonspecific complications

    (i)   Herpes labialis
    (ii) Paralytic ileus
    (iii) Jaundice
    (iv) Shock
    (v) Cardiac failure, sometimes with arrhythmia
    (vi) Deep vein thrombosis

TUBERCULOSIS

(A) Primary TB

Occurs in subjects never previously exposed to TB
'Primary complex' = Ghon focus + regional lymphadenopathy
Abdominal primary TB and tuberculous cervical lymphadenitis
are now very uncommon in the United Kingdom

Pulmonary primary TB : Usually heals spontaneously

Complications
1. Local spread in lung
2. Cavitation
3. Pleural effusion
4. Rupture of caseous node into bronchus causing widespread bronchopneumonia
5. Segmental collapse due to bronchial compression by nodes
6. 'Middle lobe syndrome', i.e. bronchiectasis in later life due to bronchial compression by nodes
7. Haematogenous metastasis
     Bone
     Kidney
     Epididymis or Fallopian tubes
     Meninges.
8. Miliary TB

(B) Post-Primary TB

Reinfection or recrudescence of primary lesion
Usually pulmonary

Complications of pulmonary TB
1. Caseation ('cold abscess')
2. Bronchogenic spread in lungs
3. Pleurisy
4. Effusion or TB empyema
5. Haemoptysis, may be massive
6. Tension cavity due to valvular obstruction
7. Tuberculoma of lungs
8. Haematogenous metastasis or miliary TB
9. Chronic pulmonary fibrosis and compensatory emphysema (especially in miners)
10. TB tracheitis, laryngitis or stomatitis due to expectoration of mycobacteria
11. Swallowed sputum may cause intestinal TB (usually in lymphoid patches)
12. Amyloidosis

Common presentations of pulmonary TB

1. Asymptomatic (screening CXR)
2. Persistent cough
3. Tiredness, malaise, recurrent coryza, weight loss or fever
4. Pneumonia
5. Haemoptysis
6. Dyspepsia

   Note increased incidence in diabetics, patients taking steroids and after gastrectomy for peptic ulcer

DEFINITIONS OF COMMON PULMONARY DISEASES

Simple chronic bronchitis

Chronic or recurrent increase in the volume of mucoid bronchial secretion sufficient to cause expectoration

Chronic obstructive bronchitis

Chronic bronchitis in which there is persistent widespread narrowing of the intra-pulmonary airways, at least on expiration, causing increased resistance to air flow

Asthma

Is characterized by variable, often paroxysmal, dyspnoea due to widespread narrowing of the bronchioles

Emphysema

Is characterized by enlargement of the air spaces distal to the terminal bronchioles, with destruction of the alveolar walls

Causes of emphysema

Localized
1. Congenital
2. Compensatory, due to lung collapse, scarring or resection
3. Partial bronchial occlusion

   (i)   foreign body
   (ii) neoplasm
   (iii) peribronchial lymphadenopathy

4. Rarely unilateral emphysema due to bronchiolitis before age 8 years (Macleod's syndrome)

Generalized
1. Idiopathic ('primary')
2. Secondary to chronic bronchitis,⎫
                 chronic asthma,⎬usually centrilobular
                 or pneumoconiosis⎭
3. Senile (physiological)
4. Rarely familial (some due to α_1 anti-trypsin deficiency)

Chest X-rays

Causes of whole lung opacity
1. Consolidation of L lung

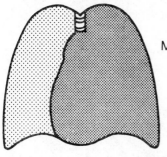

Mediastinum central

2. Massive L pleural effusion

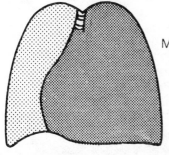

Mediastinum and trachea move to R

3. Collapse of entire L lung

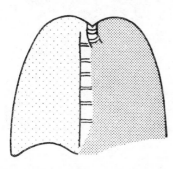

Features:
1. Trachea pulled to L
2. R heart border not seen
3. L diaphragm obscured
4. R lung hypertranslucent

Collapse of R upper lobe

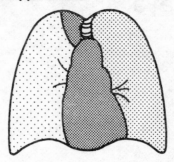

Features:
1. Dense wedge against superior mediastinum
2. R hilar vessels drawn up, and widely spaced
3. R lower and middle lobes hypertranslucent
4. Trachea and aortic knob pulled to R

Collapse of L lower lobe

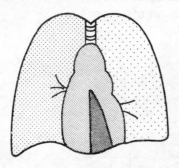

Features:
1. Dense wedge in heart shadow
2. L hilar vessels pulled down and widely spaced
3. L upper lobe hypertranslucent

R pleural effusion

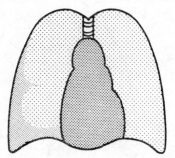

Note fluid in horizontal fissure

R hydropneumothorax

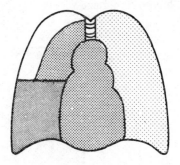

Usually traumatic

Pulmonary oedema

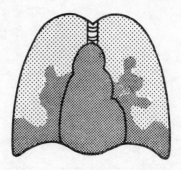

Features:
1. 'Bats-wing' shadows—ill defined and confluent spreading out from hila
2. Generalized lower-zone haze

Emphysema

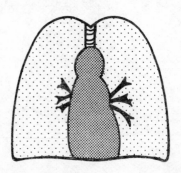

Features:
1. Hypertranslucent lung fields
2. Main pulmonary vessels are large, but peripheral vessels are thin
3. Thin vertical heart
4. Horizontal ribs with low flat diaphragm

Single large oval shadow

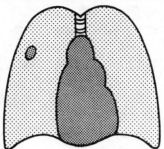

Common causes:
1. Bronchial cancer
2. Metastatic deposit, e.g. hypernephroma

Less common causes:
3. Bronchial adenoma
4. Fibroma
5. Cyst
6. Abscess
7. AV aneurysm
8. TB
9. Hamartoma

Multiple circular shadows

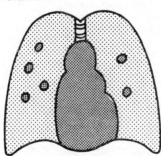

Causes:
1. Metastatic malignancy
2. Hydatid cysts
3 Caplan's syndrome (Rheumatoid arthritis with pneumoconiosis)

Widespread miliary densities

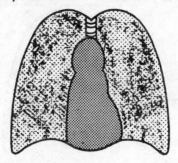

Causes include:
1. Miliary TB
2. Pulmonary oedema
3. Bronchopneumonia
4. Pneumoconiosis or haemosiderosis
5. Sarcoidosis
6. Systemic sclerosis
7. Fibrosing alveolitis and rheumatoid lung
8. Hypersensitivity, e.g. 'farmer's lung'
9. Neoplasm—Miliary Ca metastases
           Lymphangitis carcinomatosa
           Alveolar cell carcinoma

Bilateral hilar lymphadenopathy

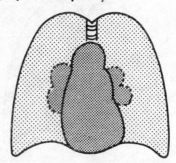

Causes include:
1. Sarcoidosis
2. Lymphatic leukaemia
3. Reticulosis
4. Carcinoma metastases
5. Primary tuberculosis
6. Acute infections, e.g. infectious mononucleosis or
   whooping-cough
   If unilateral, examine lung fields carefully for bronchial
carcinoma or Ghon focus

Normal cardiac shadow in PA X-ray

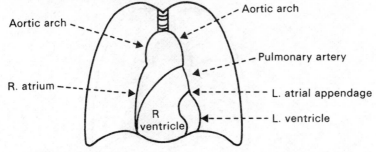

Left atrial enlargement is best seen on R anterior oblique view
Transverse diameter of heart does not normally exceed
50 per cent of chest width

Systemic hypertension

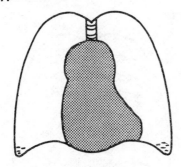

Features:
1. Aortic unfolding
2. LV hypertrophy
3. Kerley B lines (Horizontal lines in costo-phrenic angles due to
   dilated subpleural lymphatics) if LV failure develops

Mitral stenosis

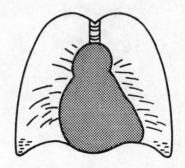

Features:
1. Straight L heart border and convex R border
2. Increased pulmonary vascular shadows
3. Kerley B lines

Coarctation of aorta

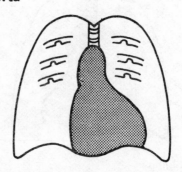

Features:
1. LV hypertrophy
2. Small aortic arch
3. Rib notching

Pericardial effusion

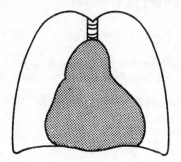

Features:
1. Large rounded heart shadow
2. Note sharp cardio-phrenic angles
Distinction from dilated heart may be very difficult

Gastro-enterology

Causes of atrophic glossitis (*smooth red tongue*)
1. Antibiotics
2. Anaemia due to deficiency of Fe, B_{12} or folate
3. Vitamin deficiency (riboflavin or nicotinic acid)

Common causes of severe upper GI bleeding
1. Duodenal ulcer
2. Oesophageal varices
3. Erosive gastritis
4. Gastric ulcer
5. Erosive oesophagitis

Common causes of severe lower GI bleeding
1. Ulcerative colitis
2. Carcinoma of rectum or colon
3. Benign rectal polyps
4. Haemorrhoids or anal fissure
5. Rectal trauma, including biopsy

CAUSES OF DYSPHAGIA

1. **Lesions of mouth or pharynx**
    (i) Stomatitis or glossitis
    (ii) Tonsillitis
    (iii) Quinsy, retropharyngeal abscess
    (iv) Lymphoma of tonsil

2. **Foreign body in pharynx or oesophagus**

3. **Intrinsic disease of pharynx or oesophagus**
    (i) Plummer-Vinson syndrome—Iron deficiency, glossitis, pharyngeal web and koilonychia
    (ii) Pharyngeal pouch
    (iii) Inflammation, stricture or neoplasm of oesophagus
    (iv) Systemic sclerosis
    (v) Oesophageal achalasia

4. **Extrinsic compression**
    (i) Tumours in neck
    (ii) Mediastinal tumour, e.g. retrosternal goitre, lymph nodes
    (iii) Bronchial cancer
    (iv) Aortic aneurysm

5. **CNS lesions**
    (i) Bulbar or pseudo-bulbar palsy
    (ii) Myasthenia gravis
    (iii) Congenital muscular incoordination

PEPTIC ULCERS
Differences between gastric and duodenal ulcers

	Gastric	Duodenal
Site	Usually middle 2/3 of lesser curve	Usually duodenal bulb
Gastric acid	Low or normal	Hyperchlorhydria
Pain	After meals	Relieved by meals May occur at about 2 a.m.
Vomiting	Common	Uncommon
Sex	Equal prevalence	4 x as common in men
Social class	Commoner in lower social classes	Equal prevalence
Pathology	May be benign or malignant	Virtually never malignant

Factors suggesting a gastric ulcer is malignant
Symptoms
1. Anorexia and weight loss
2. Epigastric pain not related to food
3. Dysphagia

Signs
1. Epigastric mass
2. Metastases. Look especially for

    (i)   Large irregular liver
    (ii) Supraclavicular nodes
    (iii) Deep vein thrombosis of leg
    (iv) Ascites
    (v) Krukenberg tumour of ovary (felt PR)

Barium meal
1. Filling defect and failure of peristalsis in a site other than middle 2/3 of lesser curve
2. Very large ulcer anywhere in the stomach
3. Leather-bottle stomach

   If in doubt gastroscopy and gastric cytology may help

Complications of peptic ulcer
1. Bleeding
2. Penetration, e.g. into pancreas, liver or retroperitoneal space
3. Perforation
4. Obstruction
    (i) Oedema and spasm—reversible
    (ii) Cicatricial stenosis—irreversible
5. 'Milk-alkali syndrome'—alkalosis and calcinosis, due to excessive ingestion of milk, alkali and calcium salts

CAUSES OF MALABSORPTION

1. Inadequate digestion

(i)   Gastric or intestinal resection
(ii) Hepatic or biliary tract obstruction
(iii) Pancreatic insufficiency (especially fibrocystic disease)

2. Parasites or change in intestinal flora

(i)   Tape worms
(ii) Blind-loop syndromes

3. Intestinal hurry or fistulae

4. Coeliac syndrome

(i)   Coeliac disease
(ii) Idiopathic steatorrhoea
(iii) Dermatitis herpetiformis

5. Tropical sprue

6. Intestinal infiltration

(i)   TB
(ii) Reticulosis, leukaemia
(iii) Systemic sclerosis
(iv) Intestinal lipodystrophy (Whipple's disease)

7. Enzyme defects

(i)   Disaccharidase deficiency
(ii) Hartnup disease

8. Chronic intestinal ischaemia e.g. atheroma

Clinical features of idiopathic steatorrhoea (adult coeliac syndrome)

1. Loose stools which may or may not be bulky, pale and foul-smelling
2. Weight loss (fat and protein deficiency)
3. Oedema (protein deficiency)
4. Flatulence with distended abdomen (impaired disaccharide hydrolysis)
5. Hypochromic anaemia (Fe deficiency)
6. Macrocytic anaemia (folate or B_{12} deficiency)
7. Peripheral neuritis (B-complex deficiency)
8. Glossitis and stomatitis (B-complex deficiency)
9. Osteomalacia (Ca and vitamin D deficiency)
10. Paraesthesiae, tetany (Ca or Mg deficiency)
11. Haemorrhage (vitamin K deficiency)
12. Muscle flaccidity, arrhythmias (potassium deficiency)
13. Weakness and hypotension (water and electrolyte deficiency)
14. Clubbing

CAUSES OF ASCITES

1. Carcinoma, especially ovarian or alimentary
2. Cirrhosis
3. Hypoalbuminaemia, e.g. nephrotic syndrome
4. Constrictive pericarditis, congestive heart failure
5. Thrombosis or obstruction of inferior vena cava
6. Tuberculous peritonitis
7. Peritonitis in late stages
8. Chylous ascites due to lymphatic obstruction

CAUSES OF OBSTRUCTION OF THE SMALL INTESTINE

The commonest causes are adhesions secondary to operation and bowel incarceration in an internal or external hernia

(A) Mechanical

1. Compression from without:
   Adhesions
   Fibrous bands
   Tumours, especially of female pelvic organs
2. Hernia
3. Strictures:
   Congenital atresia
   Acquired:
     Inflammatory
     Neoplastic
     Traumatic
4. Obturation:
   Gallstones
   Faecal impaction
   Meconium ileus
   Foreign bodies
   Worms
5. Volvulus
6. Intussusception

(B) Paralytic Ileus

1. Abdominal surgery
2. Peritonitis
3. Acute systemic illness, e.g. pneumonia
4. Painful lumbar conditions, e.g. renal colic,
                              retroperitoneal haematoma
5. Mesenteric ischaemia
6. Drugs, e.g. ganglion-blockers
7. Hypokalaemia

c

MEDICAL CAUSES OF ACUTE ABDOMINAL PAIN
Common causes
1. Food poisoning or dietary indiscretion
2. Peptic ulcer, gastritis, oesophagitis
3. Biliary colic or cholecystitis
4. Pancreatitis
5. Hepatic congestion (hepatitis, cardiac failure)
6. Renal colic, pyelonephritis or cystitis
7. Diverticulitis, ulcerative colitis, regional ileitis
8. Mesenteric adenitis (children)
9. Mesenteric ischaemia (atheroma, embolism, polyarteritis nodosa)
10. Aortic dissection
11. Gynaecological, e.g.
    Mittelschmerz (ovulation)
    Dysmenorrhoea
    Salpingitis
    Threatened abortion
12. Pain referred from spine or chest

N.B. Pain in the abdomen which lasts for more than 6 hours without remission is likely to be surgical

CAUSES OF HEPATOMEGALY
1. Hepatic congestion, e.g. cardiac failure
                          hepatic vein thrombosis
2. Neoplasm
    (i)   Metastases
    (ii) Lymphoma
    (iii) Hepatoma
3. Myeloproliferative disease, e.g. leukaemia
                                    myelofibrosis
4. Infective
    (i)   Viral, e.g. hepatitis
    (ii) Bacterial, e.g. Weil's disease
    (iii) Protozoal, e.g. amoebic abscess
    (iv) Parasitic, e.g. hydatid cyst
5. Biliary obstruction
6. Fatty infiltration or early cirrhosis
7. Storage disorders, e.g. amyloidosis
                          Gaucher's

REGIONAL ILEITIS (CROHN'S DISEASE)
Clinical features
1. Usually young adults
2. Malaise, weakness, weight loss, pyrexia
3. Intermittent colicky pain in R iliac fossa
4. Mild or moderate diarrhoea
5. Tenderness in R iliac fossa, sometimes with a fixed mass

Complications
1. Obstruction due to stricture
2. Perforation
3. Abscess
4. Fistula into anus, bladder or abdominal wall
5. Fissure-in-ano
6. Malabsorption (especially B_{12})
7. Procto-colitis
8. Erythema nodosum
9. Clubbing

Ba studies (may need both meal and enema)
1. Luminal narrowing of ileum (Kantor's 'string sign')
2. Distorted mucosal pattern
3. 'Skip' lesions

The correlation between radiological appearance and disease activity is often poor

DIVERTICULITIS
Clinical features
1. Usually middle-aged or elderly
2. Recurrent bouts of colicky abdominal pain
3. Nausea and vomiting
4. May be either constipation or diarrhoea
5. Tenderness in L iliac fossa, sometimes with a mass

Complications
1. Obstruction due to stricture
2. Perforation
3. Abscess
4. Fistula into bladder or vagina

Ba enema
1. Diverticula may or may not be seen
2. Segmental spasm and irritability of the affected colon (usually sigmoid)
3. Chronic fibrotic deformity

ULCERATIVE COLITIS
Clinical features
1. Commonly presents in 3rd or 4th decade
2. Malaise, weakness, weight loss, pyrexia
3. Chronic diarrhoea, with blood and mucus, which is often severe
4. Pain in L iliac fossa, and rectal tenesmus

Complications
1. Perforation
2. Perianal abscess
3. Acute 'toxic dilatation'
4. Severe haemorrhage
5. Hypokalaemia, hypoproteinaemia, dehydration
6. Skin lesions:
    (i) Pyoderma gangrenosum
    (ii) Aphthous ulcers
    (iii) Erythema nodosum
    (iv) Clubbing
7. Diffuse liver disease
8. Arthritis and uveitis
9. Amyloidosis after chronic abscesses
10. Carcinoma of colon

Ba enema
1. Loss of haustration
2. Straight, narrow, inelastic colon
3. May be 'spicules' due to tiny ulcer craters
4. May be filling defects due to 'pseudopolyps'

CIRRHOSIS
Cirrhosis is characterized by hepatic parenchymal damage with fibrosis and nodular regeneration throughout the liver, accompanied by distortion of the normal lobular pattern

Causes of cirrhosis
1. Cryptogenic (idiopathic)
2. Alcoholism
3. Viral hepatitis (especially serum hepatitis)
4. 'Auto-immune' liver disease
    Primary biliary cirrhosis (Hanot)
    Active chronic hepatitis (Lupoid hepatitis)
5. Haemochromatosis (primary or secondary)
6. Wilson's disease
7. Hepatotoxins, e.g. methotrexate, carbon tetrachloride

Conditions causing fibrosis but not true cirrhosis
1. Extrahepatic biliary obstruction
2. Chronic venous congestion (e.g. cardiac failure)
3. Schistosomiasis
4. Congenital syphilis

Clinical features of portal cirrhosis (Laennec)
(A) *Features of hepatic failure*
- (i) Firm hepatomegaly in the early stages
- (ii) Low grade fever
- (iii) Skin changes:
    Jaundice in later stages
    'Spiders'
    Palmar erythema
    White nails
- (iv) Bleeding tendency (decreased coagulation factors)
- (v) Fatigue, weight loss, dyspepsia
- (vi) Foetor hepaticus
- (vii) Encephalopathy:
    Lethargy
    Slow, slurred speech
    Flapping tremor
    Dementia
    Precoma progressing to
    delirium and coma
- (viii) Water retention:
    Oedema
    Hyponatraemia

(B) *Features of portal hypertension*
- (i) Splenomegaly, often with pancytopaenia (hypersplenism)
- (ii) GI bleeding from oesophageal varices
- (iii) Ascites (low plasma albumin is also necessary)

(C) *Other features*
- (i) Clubbing
- (ii) Hyperkinetic circulation
- (iii) Sexual changes:
    Females: Erratic menstruation and breast atrophy
    Males: Gynaecomastia, testicular atrophy and
    scanty body hair
- (iv) Parotid enlargement ⎫ in alcoholics
- (v) Dupuytren's contracture ⎭
- (vi) Susceptibility to infections

Causes of cholestasis

1. Extra-hepatic

    (i)   Stone in common bile-duct (CBD)
    (ii) Carcinoma of head of pancreas or biliary tract
    (iii) Pressure on CBD from lymph nodes
    (iv) Stricture of CBD (post-operative or post-inflammatory)
    (v) Developmental anomalies (rare)

2. Intra-hepatic

    (i)   Hepatitis
    (ii) Primary biliary cirrhosis (Hanot)
    (iii) Drugs—Hypersensitivity, e.g. chlorpromazine
                   Dose-related, e.g. methyltestosterone
    (iv) Pregnancy or oestrogen ingestion

JAUNDICE

Summary of urinary and faecal bile pigment changes

	Obstructive	Hepatocellular failure with no obstruction	Haemolytic
Urinary Bilirubin	Increased	Normal or Increased	Normal
Urinary Urobilinogen	Decreased	Normal or Increased	Increased
Faecal Stercobilinogen	Decreased	Normal	Increased

Haematology

CAUSES OF ANAEMIA
(A) Deficient RBC production
1. *Deficiency* of :
   Fe
   B_{12} or folic acid
   Vitamin C
   Protein
2. *Aplastic anaemia*
3. *Marrow infiltration:*
   Leukaemia
   Lymphoma, e.g. Hodgkin's
   Myeloma
   Myelosclerosis
   Metastatic carcinoma
4. *'Symptomatic':*
   Anaemia of chronic infection
   Uraemia
   Liver disease
   Hypothyroidism
   Hypopituitarism
   Malignancy
   Collagen-vascular disease, e.g. SLE
   Rheumatoid disease

(B) Loss or destruction of RBCs
1. *Haemorrhage*
2. *Haemolysis* (p. 64)
3. *Hypersplenism*

Some RBC abnormalities seen in a blood film
Size
Anisocytosis—variation in size, due to anaemia
Macrocytosis—seen in a film as increased diameter of RBC's, but defined as an increase in mean corpuscular *volume*
Microcytosis—defined as a decrease in mean corpuscular *volume*

(continued)

Shape

Poikilocytosis—variation in shape, due to anaemia which is usually severe

Spherocytosis—spheroidal cells seen in hereditary spherocytosis and in acquired haemolytic anaemia

Elliptocytosis—elliptical cells. Hereditary. Haemolytic anaemia may or may not occur

Sickling—crescentic cells seen when reducing agents act on Hb-S. Hereditary. Sickle-cell anaemia may or may not occur

Bizarre shapes—seen in severe uraemia and carcinomatosis

Staining

Hypochromia—decreased intensity of stain, due to Fe deficiency

Polychromasia—diffuse basophilia. Indicates active blood regeneration, just as reticulocytosis does

Punctate basophilia—stippled appearance seen in severe anaemia or lead poisoning

Target cells (Mexican hat cells) occur in:

  (i) Fe deficiency
  (ii) liver disease
  (iii) after splenectomy
  (iv) inherited Hb defect, e.g. thalassaemia

Causes of haemolytic anaemia

(A) *Congenital*
1. Spherocytosis ('acholuric jaundice')
2. Haemoglobinopathy:

  (i) sickle-cell anaemia
  (ii) thalassaemia syndromes

3. Non-spherocytic (enzyme defects)

(B) *Acquired*
1. Auto-immune haemolysins:

  (i) Idiopathic warm or cold antibodies
  (ii) Viral or mycoplasmal infection

2. Secondary (symptomatic):

  (i) Chronic lymphatic leukaemia
  (ii) Malignant lymphoma
  (iii) SLE
  (iv) Malaria
  (v) Uncommonly—
       renal disease
       liver disease
       carcinoma
       rheumatoid disease
       TB or syphilis

3. Drugs and chemicals, e.g. lead, methyldopa
4. Haemolytic disease of the newborn

Macrocytic anaemia:

Causes of folic acid deficiency

1. Dietary deficiency or malabsorption
2. Pregnancy
3. Increased cell turnover, e.g. leukaemia or reticulosis
4. Anti-folate drugs, e.g. anticonvulsants

Causes of vitamin B_{12} deficiency

1. Pernicious anaemia or gastrectomy
2. Changed intestinal flora, e.g. blind-loop syndrome
3. Ileal disease, e.g. Crohn's
4. Fish tape-worm (Diphyllobothrium latum)

Clinical features of Addisonian pernicious anaemia

1. Usually over 30, may have blue eyes, fair hair, premature greying
2. Anaemia of insidious onset
3. Glossitis, often intermittent
4. GI symptoms, e.g. dyspepsia, diarrhoea
5. Subacute combined degeneration
    (i) Peripheral neuritis
    (ii) Dorso-lateral column involvement
    (iii) Mental changes
    (iv) Rarely optic atrophy, nystagmus, impotence, etc.

    N.B. may be mixed upper motor-neurone and lower motor-neurone signs
6. Mild pyrexia
7. Slight hepato-splenomegaly
8. Retinal haemorrhage
9. Increased incidence of Ca. stomach

Causes of pancytopaenia

1. Aplastic anaemia (q.v.)
2. Acute leukaemia (in subleukaemic phase)
3. Marrow infiltration:
   - (i) Malignant lymphoma
   - (ii) Metastatic carcinoma
   - (iii) Myelomatosis
   - (iv) Myelosclerosis (in late stages)
4. Hypersplenism
5. Pernicious anaemia
6. SLE
7. Rarely, disseminated TB

Causes of neutropaenia severe enough to cause symptoms (agranulocytosis)

1. Aplastic anaemia

   - (i) Idiopathic
   - (ii) Drugs, e.g.
          cytotoxic drugs
          phenylbutazone
          chloramphenicol
   - (iii) Chemicals, e.g. benzene
   - (iv) Radiation

2. Selective drug-induced neutropaenia (normal Hb and platelets) e.g. amidopyrine and thiouracil
3. Acute leukaemia (in subleukaemic phase)
4. Hypersplenism
5. Idiopathic (rare)

Causes of neutrophil leucocytosis
1. Bacterial infections
2. Myeloproliferative disease:
   Myeloid leukaemia
   Myelosclerosis
   Polycythaemia vera
3. Haemorrhage, especially internal
4. Tissue damage:
   Trauma (including surgery)
   Burns
   Myocardial infarction
5. Malignancy, especially necrotic tumours and hepatic metastases
6. Drugs, especially steroids

Causes of eosinophilia
1. *Allergy*
   Hypersensitivity to food or drugs
2. *Parasites*
   e.g. trichiniasis, hydatid
3. *Skin disease*

   (i) Scabies
   (ii) Atopy (eczema, urticaria, hay fever, asthma)
   (iii) Dermatitis herpetiformis

4. *Pulmonary eosinophilia*
   A range of diseases characterized by radiographic pulmonary infiltrates, eosinophilia, and varying degrees of asthma and vasculitis, e.g. Löffler's disease and the pulmonary form of polyarteritis nodosa
5. *Malignancy,* especially Hodgkin's disease

Causes of polycythaemia
1. Polycythaemia vera
2. Hypoxia, e.g.
    (i)   High altitude
    (ii) Cyanotic heart disease
    (iii) Pulmonary disease
    (iv) Obesity
3. Miscellaneous causes of increased erythropoietin, e.g.
    (i)   Kidney cyst, neoplasm or hydronephrosis
    (ii) Liver carcinoma
    (iii) Cerebellar haemangioblastoma

Clinical features of polycythaemia vera
1. Headache, dizziness and lassitude
2. Plethoric appearance; engorged conjunctival and retinal vessels
3. Hypertension
4. Splenomegaly
5. Generalized pruritus
6. Dyspepsia due to GI vessel enlargement, or associated peptic ulcer
7. Thrombosis, e.g. cerebral, coronary or mesenteric
8. Haemorrhagic tendency
9. Peripheral ischaemia due to slow circulation or thrombosis
10. Gout

Causes of splenomegaly
1. *Infections* especially infectious mononucleosis, septicaemia, bacterial endocarditis and malaria
2. *Blood dyscrasis*
    (i)   Leukaemia (especially chronic myeloid)
    (ii) Haemolytic anaemia
    (iii) Myelosclerosis
    (iv) Polycythaemia vera
3. *Malignant lymphomas*
4. *Portal hypertension*
5. *Lipoid storage disease*
6. *Occasionally in rheumatoid disease and SLE*

Causes of lymphadenopathy

1. *Infections*

    (i) Focal infection with regional lymphadenopathy, e.g. sepsis, TB, primary chancre
    (ii) Infectious mononucleosis
    (iii) Rubella
    (iv) Secondary syphilis
    (v) Toxoplasmosis
    (vi) Tropical infestation, e.g. filariasis

2. *Lymphoma*

    (i) Hodgkin's
    (ii) Reticulum cell sarcoma
    (iii) Lymphosarcoma
    (iv) Giant follicular lymphoma (Brill–Symmer's disease)

3. *Leukaemia,* usually lymphatic

4. *Malignancy*

    (i) Metastases
    (ii) Reactive changes

5. *Miscellaneous*

    (i) Sarcoidosis
    (ii) Histiocytosis X
    (iii) Chronic inflammatory skin disease
    (iv) Collagen vascular disease, e.g. RA, SLE
    (v) Anticonvulsant drugs

CLINICAL FEATURES OF HODGKIN'S DISEASE

1. Weight loss, malaise, lassitude
2. Fever (the periodic pattern (Pel–Ebstein) is uncommon)
3. Large, discrete, rubbery superficial lymph nodes
4. Mediastinal or retroperitoneal node involvement
5. Hepato-splenomegaly
6. Pulmonary or pleural infiltration
7. Pain or paralysis due to pressure on nerves or spinal cord
8. Marrow infiltration with pain or pathological fracture
9. Skin:
    pruritus
    pigmentation
    herpes zoster
    nodular infiltrates
10. Infections due to decreased cell-mediated immunity
11. Alcohol-induced pain

CLINICAL FEATURES OF THE 3 COMMON LEUKAEMIAS

Anaemia, constitutional symptoms (fever, malaise, weight loss) and bleeding (including purpura) occur in all 3 types but are more severe in acute leukaemia and less severe in chronic lymphatic leukaemia

Acute leukaemia
1. Occurs at any age
2. Onset may be abrupt or insidious
3. Stomatitis and pharyngitis
4. Susceptibility to infections, especially of upper respiratory tract
5. Slight lymphadenopathy
6. Slight or moderate liver and spleen enlargement
7. Bone and joint pain, with sternal tenderness

Chronic myeloid leukaemia
1. Occurs in middle age
2. Insidious onset
3. Massive splenomegaly
4. Slight lymphadenopathy
5. Moderate hepatomegaly

Chronic lymphatic leukaemia
1. Occurs in late middle age, more often in males
2. Insidious onset, often found accidentally
3. Moderate or marked lymphadenopathy
4. Recurrent chronic infections
5. Moderate liver and spleen enlargement
6. May be haemolytic anaemia
7. Skin lesions:
    pruritus
    herpes zoster
    nodular infiltrates
    l'homme rouge

CLINICAL FEATURES OF MYELOMATOSIS

1. Progressive anaemia
2. Bone pain:
    (i) osteolytic lesions
    (ii) pathological fractures
    (iii) osteomalacia (due to renal phosphate leak)
3. Bleeding, due to thrombocytopaenia
4. Fever
5. Renal involvement:
    (i) acute or chronic uraemia
    (ii) Fanconi syndrome
6. Hepatomegaly, occasionally with jaundice
7. Hypercalcaemia
8. Hyperuricaemia
9. Amyloidosis
10. Neuropathy, with raised c.s.f. protein
11. Susceptibility to infections, due to defective antibodies

N.B. IV Pyelography may precipitate acute renal failure

BLEEDING

May be due to defects of platelets, coagulation or vessels

Causes of thrombocytopaenia

1. Idiopathic thrombocytopaenic purpura (Werlhof's ITP)
2. Causes of pancytopaenia (p. 66)
3. Drugs causing selective thrombocytopaenia, e.g. salicylates
4. Incompatible or massive blood transfusions

N.B. In thrombocytopaenia, bleeding time and capillary fragility are increased, but coagulation time is *normal*

Coagulation disorders

1. *Congenital*
(*a*) Haemophilias

    (i) Haemophilia A (VIII deficiency)
    (ii) Haemophilia B (IX deficiency, Christmas disease)
    (iii) von Willebrand's disease (vascular defect+VIII
        deficiency)
(*b*) Other congenital deficiencies
    Factors I, II, V, VII, X, XI, XII or XIII

2. *Acquired*

    (i) Vitamin K deficiency
    (ii) Liver disease
    (iii) Anticoagulant drugs
    (iv) Defibrination syndrome (consumption coagulopathy)
    (v) Acute primary fibrinolysis
    (vi) Massive transfusion of stored blood
    (vii) Circulating inhibitors of coagulation

Causes of bleeding due to small vessel defects

Congenital
1. Hereditary haemorrhagic telangiectasia (Osler–Weber–Rendu)
2. von Willebrand's disease
3. Pseudo-xanthoma elasticum

Acquired
1. *Infection* e.g. Bacterial endocarditis.
   Septicaemia, especially meningococcal
2. *Drugs* e.g. Corticosteroids, carbromal
3. *Secondary to systemic disease,* (*'Symptomatic'*)

    (i) Cushing's
    (ii) Scurvy
    (iii) Dysproteinaemia
    (iv) Polyarteritis nodosa

4. *'Allergic' Vasculitis*

    (i) Henoch–Schönlein purpura
    (ii) Cutaneous vasculitis

5. *Miscellaneous*

    (i) Simple easy bruising
    (ii) Senile purpura
    (iii) Dermatoses, e.g. eczema
    (iv) Fat embolism

Neurology

THE SENSORY SYSTEM

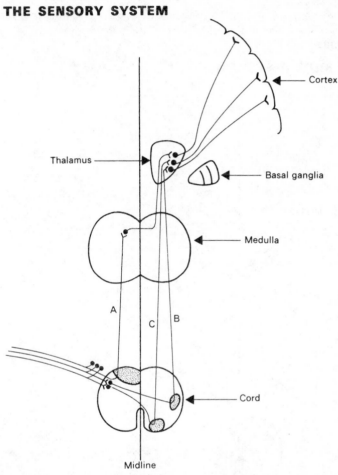

(A) *Vibration, proprioception and ½ touch fibres* travel via posterior nerve roots up the posterior column without relaying in the cord. They relay in the medulla (nuclei gracilis and cuneatus) and cross the midline to continue as the medial lemniscus to the thalamus. Tertiary fibres travel via the posterior limb of the internal capsule to the sensory cortex (post-central gyrus)
(B) *Pain and temperature fibres* relay in the cord, cross the

(continued)

midline immediately and travel in the *lateral* spinothalamic tract to the thalamus

(C) *Remainder of touch fibres* relay and cross the midline in the the cord and travel in the *anterior* spinothalamic tract to the thalamus

THE MOTOR SYSTEM

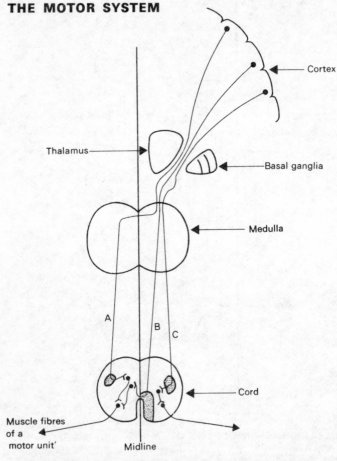

Fibres pass downwards from the motor cortex (pre-central gyrus) into the posterior limb of the internal capsule. In the pons the fibres are scattered, but they regroup in the upper medulla to form protuberances called the pyramids

    (A) In the lower medulla the majority of fibres decussate and descend in the *lateral* corticospinal (crossed pyramidal) tracts

(continued)

(B) Some fibres do not decussate, but descend in the *anterior* cortico-spinal tract, and then cross in the anterior commissure of the cord

(C) A few fibres descend directly in the *lateral* corticospinal tract with the crossed fibres from the contralateral cortex

Most fibres relay with internuncial cells in the cord, and the anterior horn cells and their fibres then form the 'final common pathway' to the motor end-plates in the muscle. The organization of movement is much more complex than this diagram suggests, since impulses are modified by the cerebellum, the extra-pyramidal system and proprioceptive and other sensations

Signs of a lower motor neurone lesion
1. Weakness and wasting
2. Hypotonicity
3. Decreased reflexes
4. Fasciculation

Signs of an upper motor neurone lesion
1. Weakness
2. Spasticity
3. Increased tendon reflexes, with clonus
4. Extensor plantar response

CRANIAL NERVE SUPPLY

1. *Olfactory* Smell
2. *Optic* Vision
3. *Oculomotor*

   (i)   All ocular muscles, except superior oblique and lateral rectus
   (ii) Ciliary muscle
   (iii) Sphincter pupillae
   (iv) Levator palpebrae superioris

4. *Trochlear* Superior oblique muscle
   N.B. Tested by asking patient to look down and *inwards*
5. *Trigeminal*

   (i) Sensory for face, cornea, sinuses, nasal mucosa, teeth, tympanic membrane and anterior two-thirds of tongue
   (ii) Motor to muscles of mastication

6. *Abducens* Lateral rectus muscle
7. *Facial*

   (i)   Motor to scalp and facial muscles of expression
   (ii) Taste in anterior two-thirds of tongue (via chorda tympani)
   (iii) Nerve to stapedius muscle

8. *Auditory* Auditory and vestibular components
9. *Glossopharyngeal*

   (i)   Sensory for posterior one-third of tongue, pharynx and middle ear
   (ii) Taste fibres for posterior one-third of tongue
   (iii) Motor to middle constrictor of pharynx and stylo-pharyngeus

10. *Vagal*

    (i) Motor to soft palate, larynx and pharynx (from nucleus ambiguus)
    (ii) Sensory and motor for heart, respiratory passages and abdominal viscera (from dorsal nucleus)

11. *Spinal Accessory*

    (i) Motor to sterno-mastoid and trapezius
    (ii) Accessory fibres to vagus

12. *Hypoglossal* Motor to tongue and hyoid bone depressors

SQUINTS
1. Concomitant squint
Due to increased tone in one ocular muscle compared with its synergist. Usually congenital, but may follow an exanthem. Occurs in all neonates.

Features

(i)   Both eyes have full movement if tested separately
(ii) No diplopia

2. Paralytic squint
Due to lesions of 3rd, 4th or 6th Cranial Nerves. Usually causes diplopia

Features

(i)   'False' image is always peripheral
(ii) 'False' image is seen by affected eye
(iii) Separation of images is maximal in direction of action of affected muscle

3rd cranial nerve (oculomotor) palsy

(i)   Marked ptosis
(ii) Eye abducted and depressed
(iii) Pupil dilated and completely non-reactive

More often partial than complete, especially with lesions near the nucleus

Cervical sympathetic paralysis (Horner's)

(ii) Mild ptosis
(ii) Enophthalmos
(iii) Pupil constricted with no reaction to shading
(iv) Reduced sweating on ipsilateral half of head and neck
(v)   Abolition of cilio-spinal reflex

Causes of Horner's syndrome

(i)   Carcinoma of apical bronchus
(ii) Cervical sympathectomy
(iii) Aortic aneurysm
(iv) Syringobulbia or syringomyelia
(v)   Brachial plexus lesions (e.g. Klumpke's paralysis)

OPTIC PATHWAY

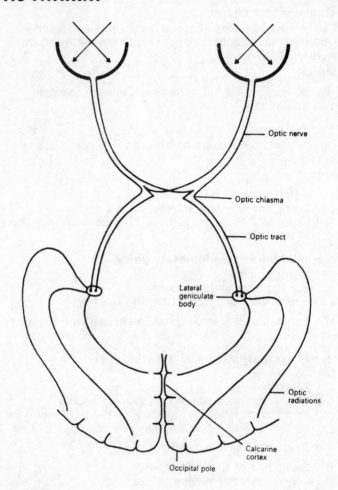

PAPILLOEDEMA
Signs of papilloedema
1. Engorged retinal veins
2. Pink disc with blurred margin
3. Loss of 'cupping'
4. Cribrosa not visible
5. Flame-shaped haemorrhages

Common causes of papilloedema
1. Arterial hypertension
2. Raised intra-cranial pressure (q.v.)
3. Retinal venous obstruction

   Papillitis (retrobulbar neuritis) is usually due to disseminated sclerosis. It resembles papilloedema but is distinguished by the early severe loss of visual acuity.

Causes of raised intra-cranial pressure
1. Intra-cranial mass or infection
2. Obstructed c.s.f flow
3. Hypertensive encephalopathy
4. Hypercapnia (CO_2 retention)
5. Pseudo-tumour cerebri
   - (i) Thrombosis of intra-cranial venous sinuses
   - (ii) Many rare causes, e.g. oral contraceptives or vitamin A poisoning

CAUSES OF FACIAL PARALYSIS
1. *Supra-nuclear* lesions e.g. cerebrovascular accident affecting internal capsule
2. *Nuclear* lesions e.g. pontine neoplasm, polio
3. *Infranuclear* lesions
   - (i) Cerebello-pontine angle and internal auditory canal, e.g. acoustic neuroma, meningioma
   - (ii) Facial canal, e.g. Bell's palsy
   - (iii) Extra-cranial, e.g. trauma, parotid neoplasm

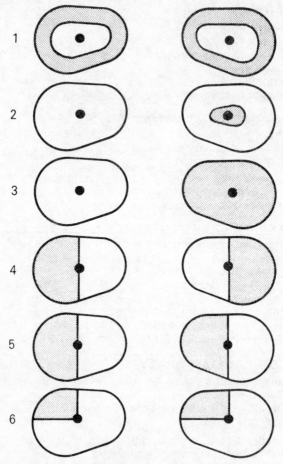

Patterns of visual field loss

1. *Concentric diminution* ('tunnel vision')
    e.g. glaucoma
2. *Central scotoma*
    e.g. retinal disease involving macula,
        retrobulbar neuritis
3. *Complete field loss in one eye*
    e.g. optic nerve lesion
4. *Bitemporal hemianopia*
    e.g. pituitary tumour
5. *Homonymous hemianopia*
    e.g. tract lesions posterior to chiasma
6. *Quadrantic hemianopia*
    e.g. temporal lobe tumours

CAUSES OF DEAFNESS.

(A) Conduction deafness

1. Wax or foreign-body
2. Eustachian obstruction
3. Otitis media
4. Otosclerosis
5. Paget's disease

(B) Nerve deafness

1. Traumatic
   Chronic exposure to loud noise
   Fractures of petrous temporal bone
2. Infective
   Congenital syphilis
   Rubella syndrome
   Mumps, influenza
3. Toxic
   Aspirin, quinine
   Antibiotics, e.g. streptomycin, neomycin
   Tobacco, alcohol
4. Degenerative
   Presbyacusis
5. Tumour, e.g. acoustic neuroma
6. Brain-stem lesions (rarely)
7. Rare familial syndromes

Rinne's test:
   The ability to hear a tuning fork through air and through
   the mastoid process are compared. In *normal* people and
   in *nerve* deafness the air conducted sound is louder,
   whereas in conduction deafness it is softer.

Weber's test:
   The base of the fork is placed on the centre of the forehead ;
   in *nerve* deafness the note is heard in the *normal* ear,
   whereas in conduction deafness it is heard in the deaf ear.

COMMON INTRACRANIAL NEOPLASMS

Children:

Medulloblastoma
Astrocytoma

Adults

Glioma
Meningioma
Metastatic cancer
Acoustic neuroma
Pituitary tumour

Clinical features of intracranial neoplasm

1. Raised intra-cranial pressure:

    (i)   Headache, worse on straining and on waking
    (ii) Drowsiness
    (iii) Bradycardia
    (iv) Vomiting
    (v) Papilloedema

2. Progressive loss of neurological function or focal neurological signs (q.v.)
3. Epilepsy
4. Mental symptoms, e.g. personality change, apathy, dementia

Localization of cortical lesions by focal neurological signs

Frontal
1. Mental disturbance: dementia
                            apathy
                            inappropriate emotion
2. Epilepsy
3. Grasp reflex
4. Unilateral anosmia
5. May be ipsilateral optic atrophy and contralateral papilloedema (Foster–Kennedy)

Pre-central
1. Jacksonian epilepsy
2. Contralateral spastic hemiplegia

Parietal
1. Sensory disturbance, e.g. lack of 2 point discrimination
2. Visual aphasia
3. Homonymous hemianopia
4. Apraxia
5. Astereognosis

Temporal
1. Anterior lesions—Motor aphasia
   Posterior lesions—Auditory aphasia
2. Homonymous hemianopia or quadrantanopia
3. Psychomotor epilepsy

Occipital
Visual field defects

Signs of a cerebellar lesion
1. Intention tremor
2. 'Scanning' speech
3. Nystagmus worse on looking to the side of the lesion
4. Limb ataxia with characteristic gait
5. Hypotonia and pendular reflexes

Causes of a cerebellar lesion
1. Disseminated sclerosis
2. Neoplasms:
    (i) In the cerebellum, e.g. medulloblastoma
    (ii) Neuropathy secondary to malignancy such as bronchial carcinoma

3. Cerebellar abscess (often secondary to otitis media)
4. Vertebro–basilar insufficiency
5. Idiopathic degeneration, e.g. primary cerebellar atrophy
6. Rare hereditary and familial ataxias, e.g. Friedreich's

SUBARACHNOID HAEMORRHAGE
Common causes
1. Ruptured 'berry' aneurysm (85 per cent)
2. Cerebral angioma (10 per cent)

Clinical features
1. Often occurs in middle life
2. Sudden onset of catastrophic headache, usually occipital. Often precipitated by straining
3. Small leakages—delirium or confusion but no loss of consciousness
   Bigger bleeds—vomiting, convulsions and coma
4. Meningism
5. Plantar responses are usually extensor
6. May be slow pulse, or hypertension
7. Occasionally squint, papilloedema, retinal haemorrhage and small sluggish pupils. The characteristic subhyaloid haemorrhage spreads out from the edge of the disc
8. May be pain in back due to blood in spinal theca

CHRONIC SUBDURAL HAEMATOMA
Cause
   Rupture of cortical veins as they cross the subdural space. May be traumatic or spontaneous

Clinical features
1. Often elderly patients, after a trivial head injury
2. Latent period of days or months occurs before symptoms develop
3. Gradual onset of headaches, memory loss, dementia, confusion, drowsiness and eventual coma. Symptoms fluctuate from day to day, with lucid intervals
4. May be signs of an intra-cranial space-occupying lesion, with localizing signs

EXTRA-DURAL HAEMATOMA
Cause
Fracture of squamous temporal bone with rupture of a branch of the middle meningeal artery

Clinical features
1. Any age, but often young adults with scalp oedema above the ear
2. Concussion may be followed by recovery of consciousness for minutes or hours before the onset of drowsiness and deepening coma
3. Signs of intra-cranial compression (p. 82)
4. Ipsilateral 3rd nerve palsy due to cerebral herniation
5. Progressive contralateral hemiplegia

The signs develop rapidly and immediate operation to relieve the pressure is mandatory

CAUSES OF CEREBRAL INFARCTION
1. Atheroma of intra- or extra-cranial arteries
2. Cerebral emboli:

    (i)   atrial fibrillation
    (ii) myocardial infarct
    (iii) bacterial endocarditis

3. Cerebral ischaemia due to severe hypotension
4. Cerebral arterial spasm, e.g. migraine or following subarachnoid haemorrhage
5. Hypoxia, e.g.
    cardiac arrest
    carbon monoxide poisoning
    pulmonary emboli
6. Arteritis, e.g. collagen vascular disease
7. Cerebral thrombosis due to polycythaemia
8. Dissecting aortic aneurysm involving the carotid artery
9. Ligation of carotid artery for intra-cranial aneurysm

CAUSES OF COMA

1. Syncope (q.v.)
2. Head injury
3. Epilepsy
4. Drugs or toxins (especially alcohol)
5. C.V.A. (Thrombosis, embolism or haemorrhage)
6. Raised intra-cranial pressure (p 79)
7. Metabolic
    (i) Hypoglycaemia
    (ii) Diabetic ketoacidaemia
    (iii) Hepatic, renal or adrenal failure
    (iv) Myxoedema
    (v) Electrolyte imbalance
8. Acute CNS infection, e.g. meningitis, encephalitis
9. Acute systemic infection, e.g. septicaemia
10. Hysteria, hypnosis
11. Hypo- or hyperthermia

SYNCOPE

A transient loss of consciousness caused by cerebral anoxia, usually due to inadequate blood flow.

Causes

1. *Vasovagal*
    (i)   Emotion, heat or standing still
    (ii) Loss of blood or plasma
    (iii) Postural hypotension, e.g. drugs or prolonged recumbency
    (iv) Carotid sinus hypersensitivity

2. *Cardiac*
    (i)   Stokes-Adams (heart block)
    (ii) Ventricular tachycardia or fibrillation
    (iii) Aortic stenosis
    (iv) Cyanotic congenital heart disease (fall in pO_2)
    (v)   Cough syncope (obstructed venous return to heart)

3. *Arterial occlusion*
    (i)   Atheroma or embolism (carotid or vertebro-basilar)
    (ii) Cervical spondylosis
    (iii) Strangulation
    (iv) 'Subclavian steal syndrome'

4. *Anoxaemia*
    (i)   High altitude
    (ii) Anaemia

ABNORMAL GAITS
N.B. Most cases are due to lesions of bone, joint or skin

'Neurological' gaits
1. *Upper motor neurone hemiplegia*
   Arm adducted and internally rotated
   Elbow flexed and pronated
   Fingers flexed
   Foot plantar-flexed, with leg swung in a lateral arc
2. *Spastic paraplegia*
   Stiff jerky 'scissors' gait, with complicated assisting movements of upper limbs
3. *Parkinsonism*
   Small shuffling hurried steps
   Flexion of neck, elbows, wrists and MP joints with thumbs adducted
4. *Cerebellar lesion*
   'Drunken' gait on a broad base. Feet raised excessively and placed carefully, with patient looking ahead. Tends to fall to side of lesion
5. *Posterior column lesion*
   Patient walks on a broad base but bangs feet down clumsily and tends to look at feet. Rombergism is present
6. *High-stepping gait*
   Due to foot drop
7. *Proximal myopathy*
   Waddling gait with broad base, lordosis and marked body swing
   This gait occurs also in congenital hip dislocation and pregnancy
8. *Hysterical*
   Usually bizarre and inconsistent, and the patient rarely falls
9. *Involuntary movements*

   (i)   *Choreiform*—Jerky movements of short duration, affecting limbs and face
   (ii) *Athetoid*—Slow writhing of arms and legs with flexed fingers, thumb and wrist
   (iii) *Dystonia musculorum* (Torsion spasm)
         Intense sustained spasm of proximal and trunk muscles may cause bizarre stepping or bowing of the trunk
   (iv) *Hemiballismus*—Unilateral forceful throwing movements which are almost continuous

CLASSIFICATION OF SPEECH DEFECTS

1. Dysphasia (disorder in use of symbols for communication whether spoken, heard, written or read)
2. Dysarthria (disorder of articulation)
3. Dysphonia (disorder of vocalization)
4. Dementia (intellectual deterioration)

Causes of dysphasia

(i) Motor—due to lesion of inferior frontal gyrus of dominant frontal lobe. (Broca's area)
(ii) Sensory—due to lesion of dominant temporo-parietal cortex

Causes of dysarthria

1. Bulbar or pseudo-bulbar palsy
2. Basal ganglia lesions
3. Cerebellar lesions
4. Weakness or paralysis of facial muscles
5. Oral lesions including loose dentures

Causes of dysphonia

1. Functional (hysteria)
2. Lesions of recurrent laryngeal nerve
3. Vocal cord lesion (infection, tumour, etc.)

SPINAL CORD COMPRESSION
Symptoms
1. Root pains occur early. Often precipitated by movement or straining
2. Progressive weakness, paraesthesiae and sensory loss
3. Sphincter disturbances occur at a late stage

Signs
1. Lower motor neurone signs at level of compression and spasticity below
2. Sensory or reflex 'level'. May be hyperaesthesia at the affected level

Causes of cord compression
1. *Vertebral*

  (i)   Metastatic cancer
  (ii) Pott's disease (TB)
  (iii) Spondylosis with disc prolapse

2. *Extra-dural*

  (i)   Abscess

3. *Intra-dural*

  (i)   Infiltration of meninges—reticulosis
                                 leukaemia
  (ii) Extra-medullary tumours—meningioma
                                neurofibroma
  (iii) Intra-medullary tumours—glioma

Causes of root lesions
1. Disc protrusion
2. Spondylosis (osteophyte)
3. Metastatic cancer

Clinical features of root lesions
1. Pain in the appropriate myotome, aggravated by straining
2. Paraesthesiae in the dermatome
3. Spinal muscle spasm, e.g. lumbar scoliosis or restriction of neck movement
4. Weakness, wasting and fasciculation of the myotome, with decreased tendon reflex

Myotomes worth remembering
C6—Biceps, brachioradialis, radial extensors of wrist
C7—Triceps, ulnar extensors of wrist, finger extensors
C8—Finger flexors
L4—Quadriceps femoris
L5—Extensor hallucis longus
S1—Plantar flexors

SYRINGOMYELIA AND SYRINGOBULBIA
Syringomyelia
Usually starts in base of posterior horn of cervical region

Clinical features
Insidious onset of
1. Weakness and wasting of small muscles of hand
2. Sensory loss in hand (pain and temperature only)
3. Trophic changes:

  (i) Cyanosis of fingers
  (ii) Ulceration and scarring
  (iii) Swollen fingers due to subcutaneous hypertrophy

4. Loss of tendon reflexes
5. Painful arm
6. Spastic paraplegia
7. Charcot joints (neck and shoulders)

Syringobulbia
Medulla may be initial site, or may be involved by upward extension from cord

Clinical features
1. Facial pain or sensory loss (Cr. 5)
2. Vertigo and nystagmus (Cr. 8)
3. Facial, palatal or laryngeal palsy (Cr. 7, 9, 10, 11)
4. Wasted tongue (Cr. 12)
5. Horner's syndrome (Sympathetic)

BULBAR PALSY
Bilateral *lower* motor neurone lesions of the bulbar nuclei (9, 10, 11 and 12 with lowermost part of 7)

Clinical features
1. Dysarthria
2. Dysphagia, especially with fluids
3. Wasted fibrillating tongue
4. Palatal paralysis

Causes
1. Motor neurone disease
2. Polio
3. Encephalitis
4. Syringobulbia

D

PSEUDO-BULBAR PALSY
Bilateral *upper* motor neurone lesions of the same nuclei

Clinical features
1. Dysarthria
2. Dysphagia
3. Spastic tongue
4. Exaggerated jaw-jerk (spastic masseters)
5. Emotional lability

Causes
1. Ischaemia of internal capsule
2. Motor neurone disease
3. Disseminated sclerosis

PERIPHERAL NEUROPATHY
Characterized by symmetrical flaccid weakness and sensory changes of 'glove and stocking' distribution

Causes of polyneuropathy
1. *Many cases are idiopathic*
2. *Drugs and chemicals*
   Isoniazid
   Lead, mercury
   Many organic chemicals
3. *Metabolic*
   Diabetes mellitus
   Amyloidosis
   Acute intermittent porphyria
4. *Deficiency states*
   B_{12} deficiency
   Alcoholism
   Beri-beri
   Pellagra
5. *Infections*
   Leprosy
   Diphtheria
   Tetanus
   Botulism
6. *Miscellaneous*
   'Acute infective polyneuritis' of Guillain-Barré
   Collagen-vascular disease, esp. polyarteritis & rheumatoid disease
   Malignancy
   Sarcoidosis
7. *Congenital*
   Rare hereditary ataxias and neuropathies

DISSEMINATED SCLEROSIS

Characterized by multiple CNS lesions scattered in time and place

Clinical features

1. Spastic weakness, usually starting in legs
2. Retrobulbar neuritis:
    Misty vision
    Painful eye movements
    Slightly swollen optic disc
    Central scotoma
3. Numbness and paraesthesiae
4. Diplopia
5. Vertigo
6. Cerebellar signs:
    Intention tremor
    Nystagmus
    'Scanning' speech
7. Sphincter disturbance and impotence
8. Euphoria or other mental change
9. Painful flexor spasms

CAUSES OF EPILEPSY

1. **Idiopathic**
2. **Focal cerebral lesions**
    (i)   Birth injury or cerebral malformation
    (ii) Tumour
    (iii) Trauma, scar, irradiation atrophy
    (iv) Vascular
            CVA
            Hypertension
    (v)   Infection
            Encephalitis or meningitis
            Abscess or tuberculoma
            Syphilis (GPI or gumma)
            Hydatid cysts or cysticercosis
    (vi) Degenerative disease, e.g. presenile dementia
3. **Metabolic**
    (i)   Pyrexia in children
    (ii) Anoxia, hypoglycaemia or hypocalcaemia
    (iii) Electrolyte imbalance, e.g. water intoxication
    (iv) Uraemia.
    (v)   Hepatic coma
    (vi) Drugs and toxins
            Lead poisoning
            Withdrawal of alcohol or barbiturates
            Nikethamide

Endocrinology

THE PITUITARY
Hypothalamic control of the anterior pituitary
Stimulating hormones
1. Thyrotrophin releasing factor (TRF)
2. Corticotrophin releasing factor (CRF)
3. Somatotrophin (GH) releasing factor (SRF)
4. Luteinising hormone releasing factor (LRF)
5. Follicle-stimulating hormone releasing factor (FRF)

Inhibiting hormones
1. Prolactin inhibiting factor (PIF)
2. Melanocyte-stimulating hormone inhibiting factor (MIF)

Clinical features of hypothalamic lesions
1. Diabetes insipidus with variable deficiencies of anterior pituitary hormones
2. Obesity
3. Somnolence
4. Variations in body temperature
5. Precocious puberty
6. Irregular menstruation

Clinical features of acromegaly
Symptoms:
1. Often insidious, with no symptoms
2. Headaches
3. Paraesthesiae (median nerve compression)
4. Weakness and joint pains
5. Polyuria
6. Impotence and loss of libido in men
7. Hirsutism and amenorrhoea in women
8. Visual deterioration
9. Galactorrhoea

(continued)

Signs:
1. Characteristic facies, large hands and feet
2. Leathery furrowed skin. May be seborrhoea, hyperhidrosis or pigmentation
3. Hoarse deep voice
4. Nontoxic goitre
5. Progressive kyphosis
6. Bitemporal hemianopia, optic atrophy, ocular palsies
7. Generalized splanchnomegaly
8. Cardiac failure (hypertension and ischaemia)
9. Signs of diabetes mellitus or its complications
10. Hypopituitarism
11. Thyrotoxicosis

Causes of hypopituitarism

1. Tumours:
    Eosinophil adenoma
    Chromophobe adenoma
    Craniopharyngioma
    Metastatic cancer
2. Iatrogenic—hypophysectomy or irradiation
3. Pituitary necrosis due to ante- or post-partum haemorrhage (Sheehan's syndrome)
4. Granulomatous infiltration, e.g. sarcoidosis
5. Trauma
6. Infection, e.g. TB meningitis

Clinical features of hypopituitarism

Loss of anterior pituitary hormones is usually partial, in the following order of frequency:

1. *Somatotrophin (GH):*
    Dwarfism in children
    Insulin sensitivity in adults
2. *Prolactin:*
    Failure of lactation in post-partum patients
3. *Gonadotrophins:*
    Delayed puberty in children
    Loss of body hair, fine wrinkled skin, impotence, infertility and amenorrhoea in adults
4. *Thyrotrophin (TSH):*
    Hypothyroidism
5. *Corticotrophin (ACTH):*
    Hypoadrenalism (asthenia, nausea, vomiting, hypoglycaemia, collapse)
6. *Melanocyte-stimulating hormone (MSH):*
    Skin pallor

THE THYROID
Causes of hypothyroidism
(A) *Primary (Thyroid gland failure)*
   1. Autoimmune thyroiditis
       Hashimoto's disease and its atrophic variant, myxoedema.
       In Hashimoto's the thyroid is large and may be tender, but
       in myxoedema it is impalpable. Circulating thyroid
       antibodies occur in both
   2. Iatrogenic:
       Surgery
       Irradiation
       Antithyroid drugs
   3. Endemic cretinism (maternal iodine deficiency)
   4. Absence or maldevelopment of thyroid gland (rare)
   5. Dyshormonogenesis (rare congenital enzyme defects
       affecting hormone synthesis)
(B) *Secondary (TSH deficiency)*
   1. Pituitary lesion
   2. Rarely hypothalamic lesion (due to thyrotrophin releasing
       factor deficiency)

Clinical features of hypothyroidism
1. Mental and physical sluggishness
2. Cold intolerance
3. Constipation
4. Weight gain
5. Croaking voice, with slow speech
6. Rough, dry yellowish skin
7. 'Myxoedema facies' with generalized thickening of
    subcutaneous tissue, periorbital puffiness, brittle sparse hair
    and thin eyebrows
8. Bradycardia
9. Delayed relaxation of tendon jerks

Less commonly—
10. Anaemia
11. Cyanosis, Raynaud's phenomenon or angina
12. Carpal tunnel syndrome
13. Perceptive deafness
14. Myalgia or arthralgia
15. 'Myxoedema madness'
16. Coma

Causes of 'non-toxic' goitre

1. 'Simple' colloid goitre (idiopathic), common during puberty and pregnancy
2. Iodine deficiency
3. Goitrogens, e.g. antithyroid drugs, excess iodine
4. Auto-immune thyroiditis (Hashimoto's)

Possibility of malignancy is suggested by:
1. Asymmetrical enlargement with 'cold area' on scan
2. Very hard thyroid
3. Pressure effects, e.g. hoarseness
4. Cervical lymphadenopathy

Causes of hyperthyroidism

1. Graves' disease
2. Toxic multinodular goitre. Resembles Graves' disease but patients tend to be older, with fewer eye signs
3. Toxic adenoma
4. Iatrogenic (excess thyroid hormone)

Clinical features of Graves' disease

Thyroid gland
1. Goitre, usually diffuse (but may be nodular)
2. Increased thyroid vascularity (thrill, bruit)

Metabolic
3. Increased heat production (warm moist skin, heat intolerance)
4. Weight loss, increased appetite, diarrhoea
5. Tachycardia, exertional dyspnoea, hyperdynamic circulation
6. Tiredness, irritability, nervousness
7. Fine tremor, hyperkinesia
8. Proximal muscle weakness with hyperactive reflexes
9. Occasionally, bone pain due to osteoporosis
10. In elderly patients, atrial fibrillation or cardiac failure

Extra-thyroid manifestations (possibly immunological)
11. Eye signs :
    Eyelid oedema
    Conjunctivitis
    Exophthalmos
    Lid retraction or lag
    Ophthalmoplegia (usually superior rectus)
12. Pretibial myxoedema
13. Thyroid acropachy (clubbing)
14. Vitiligo
15. Splenomegaly

Management of thyrotoxicosis

1. *Indications for thyroidectomy*

  (i)   Possible malignancy
  (ii) Pressure symptoms
  (iii) Retrosternal goitre
  (iv) Large goitre
  (v)   Refusal or failure of medical treatment
  (vi) Hypersensitivity to antithyroid drugs

2. *Indications for medical treatment*

  (i)   Children
  (ii) Pregnancy
  (iii) Mild hyperthyroidism with small goitre
  (iv) Patients unsuitable for surgery

3. *Indications for radio-iodine therapy*

  (i)   Relapse after thyroidectomy
  (ii) Patients over age 45

Subsequent hypothyroidism is common (about 40 per cent at 10 years)

THE PARATHYROIDS

Causes of hyperparathyroidism

1. *Primary:*
   Adenoma (85 per cent)
   Hyperplasia
   Carcinoma
2. *Secondary*
   Hyperplasia due to chronic renal failure, osteomalacia or rickets
3. *Tertiary:*
   A development of secondary parathyroidism in which the glands become autonomous

Clinical features of hyperparathyroidism

1. Due to hypercalcaemia

(i)   Anorexia, nausea and vomiting
(ii) Constipation
(iii) Polydipsia and polyuria
(iv) Lethargy progressing to coma and convulsions

2. Visceral calcification

(i)   Renal calculi
(ii) Nephrocalcinosis
(iii) Conjunctival deposits and keratopathy

3. Bone resorption

(i)   Pain and deformity
(ii) Pathological fractures

4. Rarely

(i)   peptic ulcer
(ii) pancreatitis
(iii) multiple endocrine adenomatosis
(iv) pseudo-gout
(v)   Zollinger–Ellison syndrome (pancreatic adenomas, gastric HCl and pepsin overproduction with recurrent gut ulceration)

Causes of hypoparathyroidism

1. Post-operative (e.g. thyroidectomy)
2. Idiopathic (possibly autoimmune)
3. Neonatal (transient, but dangerous)

Clinical features of hypoparathyroidism

1. Due to hypocalcaemia

(i)   Tetany (paraesthesiae, stridor, cramps, hyperreflexia)
      Trousseau's and Chvostek's signs are present
(ii) Convulsions (especially in children)
(iii) Cataracts

2. In idiopathic hypoparathyroidism

(i)   Mental subnormality
(ii) Dry skin, sparse hair, poor teeth, nail dystrophy often with Candidiasis
(iii) Papilloedema and calcified basal ganglia (mimics brain tumour)
(iv) Other auto-immune disorders, e.g.
      hypoadrenalism
      pernicious anaemia

CUSHING'S SYNDROME
Clinical features
1. Obesity of trunk and face with 'buffalo hump'
2. Hypertension
3. Skin changes:
     Striae
     Bruising
     Hirsutism
     Pigmentation
4. Osteoporosis
5. Proximal myopathy
6. Menstrual disturbances
7. Neurosis or psychosis
8. Facial plethora due to polycythaemia

Laboratory features
1. Increased plasma 11−hydroxycorticosteroids ('cortisol')
     Normal values—

9 a.m.	12 midnight
7–25 μg/100ml	3–7 μg/100ml

     Loss of diurnal rhythm occurs early in Cushing's syndrome
     (i.e. midnight samples give increased value)
2. Polycythaemia with leucocytosis and eosinophil decrease
3. Hypokalaemia, with sodium in upper normal range
4. 'Diabetic' glucose tolerance test
5. 24 hour urinary 'free 11-hydroxycorticosteroids' increased

   Low dosage dexamethasone (0·5 mg q.d.s. for 2 days) causes little suppression in Cushing's syndrome
   High dosage dexamethasone (2 mg q.d.s. for 2 days) causes suppression in adrenal hyperplasia, but has little or no effect in adrenal adenoma or carcinoma, or ectopic ACTH secretion due to extra-adrenal carcinoma

CAUSES OF HYPOADRENALISM
Acute
1. Stress occurring in patients with chronic hypoadrenalism
2. Septicaemia, especially meningococcal
3. Surgical adrenalectomy, e.g. for breast cancer

Chronic
(A) *Primary*
     1. Auto-immune adrenalitis (Addison's)
     2. TB
     3. Metastatic cancer deposits occur commonly, but rarely cause hypoadrenalism
(B) *Secondary (ACTH deficiency)*
     1. Pituitary or hypothalamic disease
     2. Prolonged corticosteroid therapy

Clinical features of chronic hypoadrenalism
1. Pigmentation, especially in exposed skin, mouth, areolae, palmar creases and pressure areas
2. Debility and tiredness
3. Nausea, vomiting, weight loss, abdominal pain, diarrhoea
4. Hypotension, with low-volume pulse
5. Hypoglycaemia, especially reactive after a meal
6. Loss of body hair in women
7. Depression

Laboratory features of hypoadrenalism
1. Plasma 11-hydroxycorticosteroids may be normal or low, but fail to respond adequately to 250 μg Synacthen IM (should rise by more than 7 μg/100 ml at 30 minutes)
2. Slow excretion of a water load
3. Low plasma sodium and chloride, with raised potassium and urea
4. Low voltage ECG with flat T waves
5. Low blood sugar

DIABETES MELLITUS
Differences between the 2 main types of diabetes mellitus

'Juvenile'	'Maturity onset'
1. Thin	Obese
2. Young	Middle-aged or elderly
3. Tendency to ketosis	Resistant to ketosis
4. Low insulin secretion	Normal or increased insulin secretion
5. Sensitive to insulin	Insulin resistant
6. Require treatment with insulin	Respond to diet, and oral hypoglycaemic drugs

Differences between 'diabetic' and hypoglycaemic coma

Ketoacidaemic coma	Hypoglycaemic coma
1. Preceded by infection or insulin underdosage	Preceded by exercise, missed meal or insulin overdosage
2. Onset over hours or days	Onset in minutes
3. Deep rapid breathing	Stertorous breathing
4. Dehydration	Normal hydration
5. Sweating absent	Sweating marked
6. CNS changes unusual	CNS changes common, especially Babinski response
7. Urine—usually glycosuria and ketonuria	Urine not helpful

Complications of diabetes mellitus

1. *Ocular*

   (i) Blurred vision due to fluctuations in blood sugar
   (ii) Cataracts
   (iii) Retinopathy:
         Venous engorgement
         Capillary microaneurysms
         'Blot' haemorrhages
         'Waxy' exudates
         Retinitis proliferans
         Retinal detachment
         Vitreous haemorrhage and fibrosis
   (iv) Rubeosis iridis (new blood vessels over iris)—may
        cause glaucoma

2. *Neurological*

   (i) Peripheral neuropathy (early sign is loss of ankle jerks
        and malleolar vibration sense)
   (ii) Mononeuritis multiplex (neuropathy of several
         peripheral or cranial nerves; often asymmetrical)
   (iii) Autonomic neuropathy:
         diarrhoea
         postural hypotension
         impotence

3. *Renal*

   (i) Pyelonephritis, sometimes with papillary necrosis.
   (ii) Glomerulonephritis
         (*a*) Kimmelstiel–Wilson (eosinophilic nodules in
              glomerular tuft)
         (*b*) Proliferative, with sclerosed basement membrane
   (iii) Atherosclerosis and hypertensive vascular changes

4. *Vascular*

Occlusion by atheroma (large vessels) or endarteritis (small
vessels) may cause ischaemia of feet, myocardium, brain or
kidneys

5. *Dermatological*

   (i) Fat atrophy or hypertrophy at insulin injection sites
   (ii) Ulcers due to neuropathy or ischaemia
   (iii) Infections, especially furuncles and Candidiasis
   (iv) Pigmented scars over shins ('diabetic dermopathy')
   (v) Xanthomata
   (vi) Necrobiosis lipoidica

6. *Systemic infections*

Incidence of TB and deep mycoses is increased

CAUSES OF DWARFISM

1. *'Constitutional'*
   Racial, familial or sporadic
2. *Nutritional*
    (i)   Starvation
    (ii) Malabsorption
    (iii) Protein loss

3. *Chromosomal defects*
    (i) Trisomies, e.g. Down's
    (ii) Turner's

4. *Skeletal defects*
    (i)   Rickets
    (ii) Achondroplasia
    (iii) Gargoylism (Hurler's)

5. *Chronic systemic disease*
    (i)   Cyanotic congenital heart disease
    (ii)   Renal failure
    (iii) Hepatic failure
    (iv)   Pulmonary disease
    (v)   Anaemia
    (vi)   Infections, e.g. TB
    (vii) Glycogen storage disease

6. *Endocrine disease*
    (i)   Sexual precocity
    (ii) Hypopituitarism
    (iii) Hypothyroidism
    (iv) Congenital adrenal hyperplasia

7. *Miscellaneous rare diseases* of unknown cause, e.g. progeria

CAUSES OF HIRSUTISM

1. 'Constitutional' (often racial or familial)
2. Stein–Leventhal syndrome (polycystic ovaries)
3. Virilizing ovarian tumours, e.g. arrhenoblastoma
4. Cushing's syndrome
5. Congenital adrenal hyperplasia (of late onset)
6. Adrenal tumours
7. Androgenic drugs
8. Cutaneous porphyria

ORAL CONTRACEPTIVES

Regimes

1. Oestrogen (mestranol or ethinyloestradiol) and progestogen in combination for cycles of 20 to 22 days
2. Oestrogen alone for 15 days, followed by a combination tablet for 7 days.
3. Progestogen alone, daily without interruption

Side-effects of oral contraceptives

1. *Symptoms due to oestrogens*
   Fluid retention, weight gain
   Nausea and vomiting
   Headache
   Tiredness and irritability
   Venous stasis in legs
   Increased menstrual loss

2. *Symptoms due to progestogens*
   Depression
   Acne
   Decreased libido, dry vagina
   Muscle cramps
   Breast discomfort
   Reduced menstrual loss

3. *Gynaecological*
   Amenorrhoea on contraceptive withdrawal
   Cervical erosion
   Vaginal Candidiasis
   Increase in size of fibroids

4. *Endocrine and metabolic*
   Abnormal carbohydrate tolerance
   Increased plasma triglycerides and cholesterol
   Abnormal liver function tests (including BSP)
   Plasma protein changes, e.g. increased transferrin
   Increased serum PBI, thyroxine and plasma cortisol
   Rarely—Hypertension
   　　　　Chloasma
   　　　　Galactorrhoea
   　　　　Gall-stones

5. *Thrombo-embolic effects*
   Increased risk of thrombosis (e.g. coronary, cerebral) or embolism (e.g. pulmonary) due to increased clotting factors and platelet stickiness

Contra-indications to oral contraceptives

1. Hepatic disease
2. Breast or cervical carcinoma
3. History of thrombosis or embolism
4. Care is required in patients with a history of epilepsy, hypertension, varicose veins, oedema or diabetes mellitus

OSTEOPOROSIS

Common causes

1. Old age
2. Immobilization
3. Glucocorticoid therapy (or Cushing's disease)
4. Rheumatoid arthritis causes localized osteoporosis

OSTEOMALACIA

Common causes

1. Deficiency of cholecalciferol (vitamin D)
   - (i)   Inadequate diet, possibly aggravated by pregnancy or lack of UV radiation
   - (ii) Malabsorption
2. Chronic renal failure

Renal disease

RENAL FAILURE
Causes of acute renal failure
(A) *Pre-renal*
1. Loss of blood, plasma or water and electrolytes
2. Hypotension with normal blood volume, e.g. myocardial infarct

(B) *Renal*
1. Acute-on-chronic failure, precipitated by renal infection or dehydration
2. 'Acute tubular necrosis' (or rarely cortical necrosis)

    (i)   Sustained hypotension
    (ii) Obstetric causes, e.g. abortion or ante-partum haemorrhage
    (iii) Septicaemia (especially Gram-negative)
    (iv) Free circulating haemoglobin
    (v) Extensive tissue damage
    (vi) Toxins, e.g. heavy metals, carbon tetrachloride

3. Primary renal disease

    (i)   Acute glomerulonephritis
    (ii) Fulminating pyelonephritis
    (iii) Acute 'collagen vascular disease'

4. Hepato-renal syndromes (including Weil's disease)

(C) *Post-renal*
Obstruction in urinary tract (p. 108)

Causes of chronic renal failure
1. Glomerulonephritis
2. Pyelonephritis or TB
3. Hypertension
4. Collagen vascular disease, especially SLE and PN
5. Metabolic:
    Diabetes mellitus
    Gout
    Chronic potassium depletion
    Chronic analgesic ingestion
    Amyloidosis
6. Obstruction in renal tract
7. Congenital:
    Polycystic kidney
    Tubular acidosis
    Fanconi syndrome

Clinical features of severe 'uraemia'

1. *Dermatological*

  (i) Pruritus
  (ii) Pallor
  (iii) Pigmentation
  (iv) Petechiae
  (v) Rarely 'urea frost'

2. *Neurological*

  (i) Mental changes (confusion, paranoia, etc.)
  (ii) Apathy and weakness
  (iii) Muscle twitching
  (iv) Coma in terminal cases
  (v) Peripheral neuropathy in chronic undialysed cases

3. *Cardiovascular*

  (i) Pericarditis
  (ii) Cardiac failure due to salt and water overload
  (iii) Hypertension
  (iv) Arrhythmia (due to hyperkalaemia)

4. *Gastro-intestinal*

  (i) Dry mouth, foetor, may be parotitis
  (ii) Anorexia, nausea and vomiting
  (iii) Hiccups
  (iv) GI tract ulceration and bleeding

5. *Genito-urinary*

  (i) In acute renal failure—oliguria (< 300 ml/24 hr)
  (ii) In chronic renal failure—polyuria with fixed urinary Specific Gravity (1·010)

6. *Respiratory*
  Hyperventilation due to acidosis

7. *Haematological*

  (i) Anaemia due to
       GI bleeding
       haemolysis
       dietary restrictions
       erythropoietin deficiency
  (ii) Bleeding tendency due to platelet dysfunction
  (iii) Susceptibility to secondary infection

(continued)

E

8. *Defects in bone and calcium metabolism*
   (i)   Osteomalacia ('renal rickets' in children)
   (ii) Secondary or tertiary hyperparathyroidism
         (osteitis fibrosa cystica)
   (iii) Patchy osteosclerosis
   (iv) Occasionally osteoporosis
   (v)   Occasionally metastatic calcification of muscles,
         blood-vessels and conjunctivae

Pathological classification of glomerulonephritis

1. *Focal glomerulonephritis*
   Increased cell proliferation affecting only *some* parts of *some*
   glomeruli
   Occurs commonly as a primary disease but also occurs
   secondary to embolic nephritis (bacterial endocarditis),
   polyarteritis nodosa, and Henoch-Schönlein purpura
2. *Proliferative*
   (Usually secondary to Group A Streptococcal infection)
   All glomeruli are affected, with swelling and increased
   number of cells. 'Crescents' occur, especially in subacute
   cases
   Electron microscopy shows deposits on the capillary basement membrane
3. *Membranous*
   Uniform thickening of capillary basement membrane
   Tubules may contain lipid
4. *Minimal lesion*
   No change on light microscopy, but there may be lipid in the
   proximal tubules
   Electron microscopy shows fusion of foot processes of the
   glomerular epithelium

Causes of nephrotic syndrome

1. Glomerulonephritis accounts for 80 per cent (usually
   membranous in adults)
2. Metabolic:
   Diabetes mellitus
   Amyloidosis
   Myelomatosis
3. SLE
4. Drugs—mercurials, penicillamine, troxidone
5. Hypersensitivity reactions (pollen, insect bites)
   N.B. Malaria is an important cause in endemic areas

Types of renal tubular dysfunction
1. *Renal disease affecting medulla,* e.g. pyelonephritis
   Impairment of urinary concentration, acidification and
   electrolyte reabsorption
2. *Renal glycosuria*
3. *'Vitamin D resistant rickets'*
   Inability to reabsorb phosphate
4. *Idiopathic hypercalcuria*
   Inability to reabsorb calcium
5. *Renal tubular acidosis*
   Inability to acidify the urine causes metabolic acidosis. Less
   calcium is bound to protein and calcium filtration is increased,
   leading to nephrocalcinosis and renal stones
6. *Cystinuria*
   Defect in reabsorption of cystine, lysine, ornithine and
   arginine
7. *Fanconi syndrome* (defect of proximal tubular function due to
   one of many possible causes)
   Defective reabsorption of glucose, phosphate and amino-acids.
   Usually proteinuria, with inability to concentrate or acidify urine.
   Adult cases may be due to renal toxins (e.g. mercury, stored
   tetracycline)
   Childhood cases are associated with cystinosis
8. *Nephrogenic diabetes insipidus*
   Impaired response to ADH

Clinical features of potassium depletion
1. Muscle weakness
2. Apathy, anorexia and confusion
3. Ileus
4. Increased cardiac excitability and digitalis toxicity
5. Thirst and polyuria
6. Renal lesions
   (i) Fanconi syndrome (q.v.)
   (ii) In severe prolonged depletion, interstitial inflammation
        and fibrosis occur

Causes of polyuria
1. Chronic renal failure
2. Diabetes mellitus
3. Compulsive water drinking
4. Diabetes insipidus
   (i) Pituitary (deficiency of ADH)
   (ii) Nephrogenic (no response to ADH)
5. Potassium depletion
6. Hypercalcaemia

Causes of haematuria

(A) *Kidney lesions*
1. Glomerulonephritis, pyelonephritis, TB
2. Trauma
3. Anticoagulant overdose, bleeding diathesis
4. Hypernephroma
5. Renal infarct (including polyarteritis nodosa)
6. Bacterial endocarditis

(B) *Renal tract lesions*
1. Papillary tumour of bladder
2. Acute cystitis (including cyclophosphamide toxicity)
3. Calculi
4. Prostatic lesions:
   hypertrophy
   cancer
   prostatitis
5. Urethral inflammation or trauma
6. TB (now rare)

Causes of urinary tract obstruction

1. Stone
2. Stricture (post-op or inflammatory)
3. Stenosis (congenital)   } occur throughout
4. Neoplasm   the urinary tract
5. Clot

6. Neuro-muscular incoordination
7. Retroperitoneal fibrosis   } ureter
8. Spread of cancer from pelvic organs

9. Prostatic enlargement or cancer
10. Retroverted gravid uterus   } bladder neck
11. Trauma of labour

12. Congenital valves   } urethra
13. Phimosis or paraphimosis

Common causes of acute retention in adults are:

Males
1. Post-operative retention
2. Prostatic lesions
3. Urethral stricture

Females
1. Trauma of labour
2. Pressure from uterus
   (fetus or fibroid)
3. Hysteria

Remember that retention may also be due to a neurological lesion such as DS, tabes or cord compression

URINARY CALCULI
Factors which predispose to urinary calculi
1. Metabolic abnormalities (q.v.)
2. Urinary tract infections
3. Urinary tract stasis
4. Foreign bodies in urinary tract
5. Geographical factors (e.g. hot climate, hard water)

Metabolic causes of urinary calculi
Calcium stones
1. Hypercalcuria (on normal diet, > 300 mg/24 hr in male or > 250 mg/24 hr in female)

  (i) Idiopathic hypercalcuria
  (ii) Hyperparathyroidism
  (iii) Vitamin D excess
  (iv) Sarcoidosis
  (v) Milk alkali syndrome
  (vi) Renal tubular acidosis
  (vii) Malignancy
  (viii) Immobilization
  (ix) Cushing's syndrome

2. Alkaline urine
3. Oxaluria

Uric acid stones
  Primary or secondary gout
  Uricosuric drugs

Cystine stones
  Cystinuria
  Fanconi syndrome with cystinosis

Xanthine stones
  Xanthinuria

NEUROLOGICAL CONTROL OF BLADDER FUNCTION
  Normal bladder capacity is 300–400 ml and larger volumes should stimulate the desire to micturate. Afferent fibres travel via parasympathetic nerves to spinal 'micturition centre' (S 2, 3, 4) and bladder contraction is initiated by parasympathetic efferents. The spinal 'micturition centre' is normally inhibited by higher motor centres, which bombard it with facilitatory impulses when micturition begins, so that the bladder empties completely

Types of dysfunction

1. *Lack of normal inhibition*
   Frequency with small volumes
   Occurs in anxiety, cold weather, etc.
2. *Atonic bladder*
   Distended bladder with overflow, but no desire to micturate
   Occurs with sensory neuropathy, e.g. diabetes mellitus, tabes dorsalis
3. *Automatic bladder*
   Bladder empties partially when volume of about 250 ml is reached, but without desire to micturate
   Occurs with cord section above S 2, 3, 4
4. *Autonomous bladder*
   Large residual urine volume, with weak uncoordinated bladder contractions but no desire to micturate
   Occurs with LMN cord lesions at S 2, 3, 4 level
   Unilateral neurological lesions may cause either frequency with small volumes or a large hypotonic bladder with residual urine after micturition

ACID-BASE BALANCE

Most of the acid produced in metabolism is eliminated via the lungs.
Henderson–Hasselbach equation

$$\text{Blood pH} = pK + \log\frac{\text{Bicarbonate}}{\text{Carbonic acid}}$$

where pK is dissociation constant of carbonic acid
Blood buffers provide short-term protection against change in pH
Kidney eliminates 'fixed' acids, e.g. sulphates which cannot be excreted by the lungs

RENAL CLEARANCE

The number of ml of plasma which contains the amount of a substance excreted in the urine in one minute is the renal clearance of that substance, i.e. $C = UV/PT$ ml
where U = concentration of substance in urine
V = volume of urine collected in time T
P = concentration of substance in plasma

Rheumatology

Patterns of polyarthropathy

Primary osteoarthrosis
Symmetrical, affecting many joints
1. Knees
2. Great toes and thumbs : MP joints
3. Fingers : terminal IP joints
4. Acromio-clavicular joints
5. Small joints of spine

Secondary osteoarthrosis
Asymmetrical, affecting weight-bearing joints

1. Knee
2. Hip
3. Intervertebral discs

Rheumatoid arthritis

1. Hands : intercarpal joints, MP joints and proximal IP joints
2. Feet : tarsal and lateral MP joints
3. Knees
4. Small joints of cervical spine and subacromial bursae

Ankylosing spondylitis

1. Spine and both sacro-iliac joints
2. Knees, shoulders, wrists

Psoriasis

1. Hands, terminal IP joints
2. Sacro-iliac joints
3. 'Rheumatoid' pattern

Reiter's

1. Ankles and all joints of feet
2. Knees
3. Hips, sacro-iliac joint and spine

Causes of a single hot red joint

1. Traumatic, e.g. sprained ankle
2. Septic arthritis
   May be secondary to penetrating injury, osteomyelitis, septicaemia, rheumatoid arthritis or osteoarthrosis
3. Gout or pseudo-gout (chondrocalcinosis or periarticular calcification)
4. Haemophilia
5. Gonococcal arthritis
6. Occasionally rheumatoid arthritis

Causes of a transient 'flitting' arthritis

1. Rheumatic fever
2. Henoch–Schönlein purpura
3. Serum sickness and drug reactions
4. SLE
5. Systemic infections:
   Bacterial endocarditis
   Rubella
   Infectious mononucleosis
   Infective hepatitis
   Mycoplasma pneumonii
   Gonococcal or meningococcal septicaemia
6. Reiter's disease
7. Occasionally, acute rheumatoid arthritis

Clinical features of polyarteritis nodosa

Usually young or middle-aged men
1. Fever, malaise, weight-loss
2. Gastro-intestinal ischaemia:
   central abdominal pain
   bleeding
3. Proteinuria and haematuria. Hypertension is common
4. Peripheral neuropathy, often painful
   Focal CNS lesions
5. Arthralgia and myalgia
6. Myocardial ischaemia
7. Skin lesions:
   nodules
   livedo reticularis
   necrosis and ulceration

N.B. Asthma, haemoptysis and pneumonitis may occur in association with eosinophilia and systemic vasculitis, but some authors regard this 'pulmonary' form as an entity distinct from polyarteritis nodosa

Clinical features of systemic lupus erythematosus

Usually young or middle-aged women
1. Fever, malaise, weight-loss
2. Arthralgia, flitting or episodic
3. Rash, classically in 'butterfly' distribution. May be erythematous, urticated or purpuric
4. Proteinuria, glomerulonephritis, nephrotic syndrome or hypertension
5. Lymphadenopathy
6. Myocarditis, endocarditis (Libman–Sacks), or pericarditis
7. Pleurisy with effusion, pneumonitis
8. Hepatomegaly and splenomegaly
9. Pancytopaenia. May be haemolysis
10. Psychosis, neuropathy or epilepsy. May be retinal exudates
11. Gastrointestinal upsets (nausea, pain, diarrhoea, etc.)
12. Raynaud's phenomenon

Dermatology

ECZEMA
Eczema is a distinctive inflammatory response of the skin, characterized histologically by spongiosis (epidermal oedema) and clinically by clustered papulo-vesicles with erythema and scaling

Many cases have a multifactorial aetiology

Types of eczema
(A) *Exogenous*
1. Primary irritant dermatitis, e.g. due to caustics, detergents or solvents
2. Allergic contact dermatitis, e.g. due to hypersensitivity to metals, rubber, medicaments, etc
3. Infective dermatitis, e.g. around infected wounds or ulcers

(B) *Endogenous*
1. Atopic dermatitis (infantile eczema)
2. Seborrhoeic dermatitis
3. Discoid eczema
4. Pompholyx—vesicles on palms or soles
5. Pityriasis alba—patches of scaly eczema which leave depigmented areas
6. Asteatotic eczema—due to excessive drying ('chapping')
7. Gravitational eczema—secondary to venous insufficiency

PSORIASIS
Distinctive morphological types
1. Nummular—discoid plaques, which may be confluent
2. Guttate—'showers' of small lesions, often post-streptococcal
3. Erythrodermic—very widespread erythema, with exfoliation
4. Generalized pustular psoriasis
5. Pustular eruptions of the hands and feet

Atypical forms are common, e.g. rupioid (conical hyperkeratosis), follicular, intertriginous, etc

'Napkin psoriasis' (psoriasiform lesions in infants) may be related to Candida infection

Blistering eruptions
Common:
1. Viral:
   Herpes simplex
   Herpes zoster—varicella
2. Impetigo
3. Scabies
4. Insect bites and papular urticaria
5. Bullous eczema and pompholyx
6. Drugs, e.g. barbiturate overdose, photosensitivity

Uncommon:
7. Erythema multiforme ⎫
8. Dermatitis herpetiformis ⎬ Sub-epidermal
9. Pemphigoid ⎪
10. Porphyria cutanea tarda ⎭
11. Pemphigus group— Intra-epidermal

Rare:
12. Congenital:
    Epidermolysis bullosa
    Ichthyosiform erythroderma
    Incontinentia pigmenti

Causes of leg ulcers
1. Venous stasis
2. Ischaemia:
   Atheroma
   Arteritis
3. Neuropathy:
   Diabetes mellitus
   Spina bifida
   Tabes dorsalis
   Leprosy (in endemic areas)
4. Rheumatoid arthritis—ulceration is multifactorial
5. Malignancy—usually squamous-cell skin carcinoma
6. Haemolytic anaemia, especially sickle-cell
7. Gumma
8. Necrobiosis lipoidica (may be diabetic)
9. Pyoderma gangrenosum—often due to ulcerative colitis

Many leg ulcers have a multifactorial aetiology, e.g. ischaemia, anaemia, stasis and infection

Causes of alopecia

1. Male-pattern baldness
2. Idiopathic diffuse alopecia of women—usually post-menopausal
3. 'Telogen effluvium'—loss of club hairs after febrile illness, surgery or parturition
4. Alopecia areata
5. Drugs:
    Cytotoxic agents
    Anticoagulants
    Dextran
    Oral contraceptives
6. Scalp infection:
    Fungi
    Pyogenic bacteria
7. Systemic disease:
    Syphilis
    Hypothyroidism
    Fe deficiency
8. Traumatic:
    Traction from rollers
    Scalping injury
    Burns
    Excessive bleaching, perming, etc.
9. Dermatoses:
    Psoriasis
    Discoid lupus erythematosus
    Lichen planus
10. Congenital—Many rare diseases, e.g. monilethrix

Causes of diffuse hyperpigmentation

1. *Congenital*

    (i) Racial or genetic
    (ii) Rarely, Fanconi's syndrome (pancytopaenia with multiple congenital defects)

2. *Physical agents*

    (i) Radiation, e.g. UVR
    (ii) Chronic rubbing, e.g. 'vagabond's itch'

3. *Post-inflammatory,* e.g. erythroderma
4. *Endocrine* (Excess ACTH or MSH)

    (i) Pregnancy, oral contraceptives
    (ii) Hypoadrenalism
    (iii) Acromegaly
    (iv) ACTH therapy or ectopic ACTH from carcinoma

5. *Metabolic*

    (i) Cachexia
    (ii) Uraemia
    (iii) Hepatic disease, especially biliary cirrhosis and Wilson's disease
    (iv) Haemochromatosis
    (v) Pellagra
    (vi) Malabsorption, especially sprue
    (vii) B_{12} or folate deficiency
    (viii) Systemic sclerosis
    (ix) Porphyria

6. *Drugs and Chemicals*

    (i) Arsenicals
    (ii) Busulphan
    (iii) Chlorpromazine
    (iv) Photodynamic agents, e.g. psoralens

7. *Pigmentation not due to melanin*

    (i) Jaundice—Yellow
    (ii) Carotenaemia—Yellow
    (iii) Mepacrine—Yellow
    (iv) Ochronosis (alkaptanuria)—Blue-black
    (v) Argyria—Grey

Some causes of a circumscribed patch of red scaly rash
1. Psoriasis
2. Eczema
3. Fixed drug eruption
4. Ringworm
5. Lichen simplex
6. Bowen's disease
7. Discoid lupus erythematosus
8. Lupus vulgaris

Some causes of widespread patches of red scaly rash
1. Psoriasis
2. Eczema
3. Pityriasis rosea
4. Pityriasis versicolor
5. Pityriasis lichenoides (acute or chronic type)
6. Resolving phase of exanthemata, e.g. measles
7. Secondary syphilis

Causes of erythema nodosum
1. Sarcoidosis
2. Streptococcal infection
3. TB
4. Sulphonamides
5. Ulcerative colitis or Crohn's disease
6. Other infections, e.g.
       Leprosy
       Systemic mycoses
       Toxoplasmosis
       Lymphogranuloma venereum

Management of medical emergencies

UNEXPECTED CARDIAC ARREST

Immediately call the 'cardiac arrest team' and give a sharp thump on the praecordium. Clear the airway, start artificial respiration (mouth-to-mouth or Ambu bag) and external cardiac compression. If the bed is sprung, move the patient to the floor

When help arrives, arrange intubation and artificial ventilation with oxygen, and obtain an ECG. Start on IV infusion and give 100 mEq of sodium bicarbonate

Fibrillation should respond to a defibrillating shock and lignocaine 100 mg IV. Adrenaline (to coarsen fine fibrillation), phenytoin, calcium chloride or bretylium tosylate may also be required

Asystole may respond to calcium chloride or isoprenaline intravenously. A pacing electrode may be inserted via the jugular vein or directly through the chest wall

Acid-base balance must be corrected under laboratory control, and mannitol infusion may be required for cerebral oedema

ACUTE PULMONARY OEDEMA

Sit the patient up in a cardiac bed, with legs dependant, and give oxygen by a high concentration mask

Give morphine 10 mg IV, frusemide 30 mg IV and aminophylline 500 mg by *slow* IV injection. If the patient has not had digoxin in the last 5 days, give 1 mg IM stat, then 0·5 mg IM 6 hourly until signs of toxicity (e.g. nausea or ectopic beats) occur

If the patient is the same after 45 minutes repeat the frusemide, morphine and aminophylline injections in half-dosage. If the patient is worse, use rotating BP cuffs on the limbs and venesect 1 pint of blood.

In desperate cases consider positive pressure ventilation.

MASSIVE PULMONARY EMBOLISM

Resuscitate the patient with external cardiac compression, oxygen administration, vasopressor drugs and correction of acidosis as necessary.

Some authors advocate a large dose of heparin (15,000 units IV) to block serotonin release from the thrombus

Subsequent therapy depends on the severity of the condition

(i)   Patients likely to die within an hour or so—bypass embolectomy (if facilities available)
(ii) Slightly less critically ill patients—streptokinase infusion
(iii) Milder cases—heparin followed by oral anticoagulants

ACUTE ANAPHYLAXIS

The 'shock' is due to:

(i)   respiratory obstruction (laryngeal oedema and severe bronchospasm)
(ii) circulatory collapse (low plasma volume due to leakage of fluid into interstitial tissues)

In anaphylaxis due to an injection or sting, apply a tourniquet to the injected part as soon as possible

Hydrocortisone 300 mg IV should be given immediately together with 0·5 ml adrenaline (1 :1000) subcutaneously. The adrenaline should not be repeated, as it may accumulate at the injection site and be absorbed rapidly when the circulation improves. Some authors also advocate an antihistamine, e.g. promethazine 50 mg IV

Resuscitation with external cardiac compression, intubation (or tracheostomy) and mechanical ventilation may be required

Restoration of plasma volume by infusion of fluid may be helpful

DIABETIC KETOACIDAEMIC COMA

No inflexible rules can be given, since individual patients vary in their requirements. Treatment must be monitored throughout by frequent biochemical analysis

1. Identify and treat the precipitating cause, e.g. infection. If no cause is apparent a broad-spectrum antibiotic may be used empirically
2. Take blood for glucose, urea and electrolytes, haematocrit and blood group, and arterial blood for Astrup (pH)
3. Give 40 to 120 units of soluble insulin, $\frac{1}{2}$ IV and $\frac{1}{2}$ IM. The dose depends on whether the patient is a new diabetic or not, the degree of dehydration and shock, the presence or absence of infection, the depth of coma and the pre-coma daily insulin requirement
4. Infuse N saline rapidly—1 litre in the first hour in a young adult, but more slowly in older patients to avoid congestive cardiac failure
   N saline should be continued more slowly thereafter, depending on the clinical and biochemical response, until blood glucose has fallen to 250–300 mg/100 ml. In severe shock blood transfusion may be needed
5. If initial pH is 7·00 or below, give 1 per cent sodium bicarbonate IV cautiously, with monitoring of plasma sodium and bicarbonate
6. If there is gastric dilatation or vomiting pass a tube and empty the stomach. Bladder catheterization may be required but is not recommended as a routine
7. Check blood glucose, bicarbonate and potassium 1 hour after the first dose of insulin, and 2 hourly thereafter. If the first post-insulin blood glucose has not fallen significantly the initial insulin dose is repeated. If the first post-insulin blood glucose is *higher* than the initial glucose, *double* the initial dose of insulin is given. Soluble insulin is given 2 hourly thereafter in a dose depending on the rate of fall of blood glucose
8. As soon as blood glucose falls significantly, add potassium chloride to the infusion, at a rate of less than 40 mEq K^+ every 4 hours. Plasma K^+ must be monitored frequently
9. When blood glucose reaches 250–300 mg/100 ml the N saline infusion is replaced with 5 per cent glucose in 1/5 N saline, 1 litre 4 hourly with added K^+ as required. At this stage a regular dose of soluble insulin is instituted

'STATUS EPILEPTICUS'

Establish an adequate airway and give oxygen

Give 2 to 15 mg diazepam (Valium) by very slow IV injection until convulsions cease. If venepuncture is impossible, give 10 mg IM. A suitable alternative is paraldehyde (5 ml into each of 2 IM sites)

For longer-term control, follow this with phenobarbitone 100 mg IM and phenytoin 300 mg IV

Take blood for glucose estimation and give 50 ml of 50 per cent glucose IV to exclude hypoglycaemia

'STATUS ASTHMATICUS'

Administer oxygen with a Ventimask (35 per cent)

Give aminophylline 250 to 500 mg by slow IV injection and hydrocortisone 300 mg IV followed by a further 200 mg every 2 hours if necessary

Check the arterial pO_2, pCO_2 and pH and assess the response to treatment by serial blood gas analysis

Dehydration will require IV fluid infusion, and since many cases are precipitated by a chest infection some authors recommend antibiotic therapy (tetracycline, ampicillin or trimethoprim sulphamethoxazole)

In very severe cases, mechanical ventilation via a tracheostomy may be required. Bronchial lavage with saline is controversial

CHOLINERGIC AND MYASTHENIC CRISIS

In myasthenia gravis, too high a dose of anticholinergic drugs may make the weakness worse (cholinergic crisis). This is easily mistaken for exacerbation of the disease (myasthenic crisis), but IV injection of 2 mg edrophonium will transiently increase the strength in myasthenic crisis. Artificial ventilation may be required

For myasthenic crisis, give neostigmine 0·5 mg IM repeated every 20 minutes as necessary

For cholinergic crisis, give pralidoxime 1 to 2 g by slow IV injection, repeated every 20 minutes as necessary

In both cases the response should be monitored with further edrophonium tests, and the muscarinic effects of anticholinesterases should be blocked by injection of atropine subcutaneously

MANAGEMENT OF ACUTE POISONING

Barbiturates

Rapidly absorbed, and stomach washout is dangerous in coma unless a cuffed endotracheal tube is used

Nurse prone and clear the airways. Respiratory failure may necessitate artificial ventilation

Circulatory failure and hypothermia should be treated with fluid replacement and careful heating

Forced diuresis should be considered for phenobarbitone

Salicylates

Absorption is slow, therefore stomach washout is advisable.

Expect complicated electrolyte disturbances which require correction under laboratory control. There may be a bleeding tendency (hypoprothrombinaemia) needing vitamin K_1

Forced diuresis is required for severe cases

Ethanol

Prevention of aspiration of vomitus is important

In severe cases gastric lavage is needed, with supportive therapy as required (artificial ventilation, etc.)

In very severe poisoning peritoneal dialysis or haemodialysis is indicated

Iron Salts

High mortality in children if untreated. Symptoms are GI irritation, dehydration and delayed damage to liver and CNS

Empty the stomach immediately by inducing vomiting and follow with gastric lavage using desferrioxamine solution (2 g in 1 litre). Leave 10 g desferrioxamine in 50 ml water in the stomach and give 2 g of desferrioxamine IM

Carbon monoxide

Remove the patient from the poisonous atmosphere, clear the airway and give artificial respiration with 100 per cent oxygen with the patient prone

After spontaneous breathing starts there may be relapse into coma due to cerebral oedema, which may require IV infusion of 500 ml of 20 per cent Mannitol

Anoxic heart or brain damage may occur

Narcotics (Morphine, etc.)

Hypoventilation should be treated with nalorphine 10 mg IV, repeated if necessary up to 50 mg according to response, but note that nalorphine overdosage also causes respiratory depression

Phenothiazines
Little disturbance of consciousness and respiratory depression, but drugs for convulsions and cardiac arrhythmias may be needed

Tricyclic antidepressives
These cause dry mouth, dilated pupils, disturbed consciousness, cardiac arrhythmias and in severe cases respiratory failure and hypotension. ECG monitoring is advisable, and pyridostigmine 1 mg subcutaneously every 30 minutes may prevent the arrhythmias

Amphetamines
These cause hyperactivity and psychosis, followed by exhaustion, convulsions, hyperthermia and coma
Barbiturates counteract the early stages and later anticonvulsants, cooling and artificial ventilation may be required

Bleaching agents
These are highly irritant. Gastric lavage is advisable, and milk and aluminium hydroxide gel should be given

Dry cleaning fluids (C Cl$_4$, etc)
If inhaled, artificial ventilation may be needed
If swallowed, gastric lavage is required
Acute hepatic and renal failure may follow

Petroleum products and paraffin (kerosene)
Gastric lavage is contraindicted because aspiration of a small amount causes pneumonitis. Absorption from the stomach is slowed by giving 250 ml of liquid paraffin

Cyanide
Speed is essential. Inject two 20 ml ampoules of 1·5 per cent Dicobalt Tetracemate (Kelocyanor) intravenously, followed by 20 ml of 50 per cent glucose
This treatment is replacing the previously recommended regime of breaking an ampoule of amyl nitrite under the patient's nose and then injecting sodium nitrite and sodium thiosulphate intravenously
Gastric lavage and artificial ventilation with oxygen are also recommended

Index